COLD PRESS JUICE BIBLE

300 Delicious, Nutritious, All-Natural Recipes for Your Masticating Juicer

LISA SUSSMAN

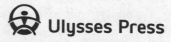 Ulysses Press

Published in the U.S. by
ULYSSES PRESS
P.O. Box 3440
Berkeley, CA 94703
www.ulyssespress.com

ISBN: 978-1-61243-393-6
Library of Congress Control Number 2014932307

10 9 8 7 6 5 4 3 2 1

Printed in Canada by Marquis Book Printing

Acquisitions Editor: Keith Riegert
Project Editor: Alice Riegert
Managing Editor: Claire Chun
Copyeditor: Renee Rutledge
Proofreader: Lauren Harrison
Front cover design: Rebecca Lown
Front cover artwork: © Anna Hoychuk/shutterstock.com
Interior design: what!design @ whatweb.com
Interior artwork: carrot © Marnikus/shutterstock.com; coconut © Marnikus/
    shutterstock.com; greens © n_eri/shutterstock.com; strawberry © n_eri/
    shutterstock.com
Layout: Lindsay Tamura
Indexer: Sayre Van Young

Distributed by Publishers Group West

NOTE TO READERS: This book has been written and published strictly for informational and educational purposes only. It is not intended to serve as medical advice or to be any form of medical treatment. You should always consult your physician before altering or changing any aspect of your medical treatment and/or undertaking a diet regimen, including the guidelines as described in this book. Do not stop or change any prescription medications without the guidance and advice of your physician. Any use of the information in this book is made on the reader's good judgment after consulting with his or her physician and is the reader's sole responsibility. This book is not intended to diagnose or treat any medical condition and is not a substitute for a physician.

To all juicers everywhere—may the green force be with you.

CONTENTS

INTRODUCTION 7

SECTION I: COLD PRESS JUICING 11

   1. The Skinny 12

   2. Setting Up Your Home Juice Bar 30

   3. Getting Juicy 43

   4. Clean Up Your Act 76

   5. Coming Clean 96

SECTION II: COLD PRESS JUICE RECIPES 121

   6. Mono Juices 126

   7. Breakfast of Champions 130

   8. Snacks 137

   9. Liquid Lunch 150

   10. Happy Hour 160

   11. Not-the-Dog's Dinner 166

   12. Sweet Course 174

   13. Late-Night Munchies 179

THE FINAL SQUEEZE 186

INDEX 189

ACKNOWLEDGMENTS 192

ABOUT THE AUTHOR 192

INTRODUCTION

The *Cold Press Juice Bible* is your essential guide to slow cold press juicing, squeezing in everything you'll need to know about getting all of the fruit and veggies your body needs—in a glass.

THIS BOOK IS FOR YOU IF...

YOU WOULD RATHER SIP A GLASS OF JUICE THAN GNAW YOUR WAY THROUGH AN OVERFLOWING BOWL OF KALE. Juicing is the easier way to get your daily nine doses of fruits and vegetables. You should be drinking about 20 pounds of produce a day. While you could have bottled vegetable juice, you don't want to. No, seriously—you really don't want to. Bottled juices may be loaded with vegetables, but the drink is usually a souped-up version of just one kind of produce, like tomato or carrot. Store-brands also tend to have more sugar (some, such as Welch's fruit juice cocktails, Jones Juice Berry White, many Arizona drinks, Minute Maid's Cranberry Apple Raspberry Juice, Fruit Works' Strawberry Melon, and Tropicana's grapefruit juices have corn syrup in their ingredient list) and more sodium (V8 measures in with almost a third of the daily recommended average adult sodium intake per serving) than a green juice made from leafy veggies like kale, spinach and chard, brassicas like broccoli and Brussels sprouts, and the odd fruit such as an apple.

YOU LIKE TO GIVE IN TO YOUR INNER HULK AND GO GREEN AND CRUSH THINGS. It's not just using a variety of green ingredients that makes juice more nutritious—the juicer you use can also amp up the health benefits. Traditional centrifugal juicers work with fast-spinning blades that heat up as they whir, exposing the produce to high temperatures and air, two things that may cut down on how many nutrients make their way into your glass. On the other hand, masticating or "cold press" juicers extract the juice by crushing and pressing fruits and vegetables without adding heat, hence the term "cold press."

YOU'RE TIRED OF FORKING OVER A HUGE CHUNK OF CHANGE FOR SOMEONE ELSE TO SQUISH FOOD FOR YOU AND PACKAGE IT IN A CUTE BOTTLE. If you're a dedicated commercial cold press juice drinker, you know that hitting up your local juice bar on a daily basis can be the cost equivalent of buying a three-course meal at a four-star restaurant. OK, the juice may also be as filling as that meal, but you can get it much more cheaply and tastily at home, and without the hipster 'tude. A cold press juicer can pay for itself in a month.

YOU WANT TO FEEL INSTANTLY BETTER THAN YOU DO RIGHT NOW. Research published in the *Journal of Environmental Science and Technology* determined that the color green (the healthiest cold press juice color) is closely linked to the environment, which can put you in a relaxed or refreshed mood.

YOU HATE TO COOK. Most cold press juicing ingredients are healthiest consumed raw (see "Raw or Cooked?" on page 49 for which produce you need to break out the saucepans for).

YOUR MOUTH IS OFTEN TIRED AT THE END OF THE DAY FROM TALKING. Drinking juice gives your jaw a rest.

YOU WANT TO STICK IT TO A SIBLING/FRIEND/CO-WORKER/NEIGHBOR/PET WHO HAS A TENDENCY TO ACT SUPERIOR TO YOU. Choosing a glass of fresh kale, parsley, sprouts, carrots, bell peppers, ginger and apple over a chocolate chip cookie is all it takes to add an instant virtuous aura to your life.

YOU'RE A SELFISH ENVIRONMENTALIST. Juicing means you help the environment while you help yourself. According to WorldWatch, around 1.6 billion gallons of oil are used each year to manufacture plastic bags and less than 10 ten percent ends up in the recycling bin (in other words, enough to drive the average gas-guzzling car around the world several tens of thousands of times if you converted the bags back to oil). But you can easily earn your green wings by taking your own bags to the supermarket or farmer's market when you stock up on ingredients. Go even greener by making compost from any leftover pulp. If you want to test how green your thumb is, you can even grow your own food for juicing and be completely sustainable in your own backyard while saving big bucks on groceries (see "Grow Your Own" on page 52).

YOU HAVE A HIGH SCHOOL REUNION/WEDDING/SEAT BOOKED ON A SPACE SHUTTLE COMING UP AND YOU NEED TO DROP SOME POUNDS FAST WITHOUT THE DIZZY DRAMA. Drinking 64 ounces of green juice daily (the typical measurement on a juice cleanse) is considerably fewer calories but more nutrients than what you'd eat on a restricted diet. Many people lose as much as six pounds on a three-day cleanse (page 108), so you'll certainly look svelte for your event. The secret to keeping it off long-term is to use the cleanse as a way to clean-slate your usual diet and continue to eat healthy and in moderation post-cleanse.

THE IDEA OF ROCKY BALBOAING YOUR WILLPOWER INTO SHAPE MAKES YOU WANT TO START SINGING, "GONNA FLY NOW." Juice cleansing gets you to challenge and test your limits (that said, the ideal time to start is not going to be your birthday or any time between Thanksgiving and New Year's Eve; however, if you must, stick with a doable one-day cleanse). Getting control over your willpower will not only give you a sense of accomplishment—it'll also have a payoff when you go back to solid food. Research from the University of Southern California shows that the self-discipline exercised in cleansing will help you stay in control in the future when a plate of nachos is calling your name—this applies even in times of stress (when healthy eating intentions are most likely to derail).

YOU WANT TO FIND YOUR ZEN. Drinking only liquids for spiritual reasons has been around for centuries. Many cultures and religions incorporate some kind of cleansing aspect to renew and rejuvenate the body, mind and soul.

Cold press juicing is the way to go. Unlike standard juices, which are heat-pasteurized, the cold press method of juice extraction slowly cold crushes and then presses the produce to preserve more of the nutrients and enzymes of whole fruits and vegetables. The result yields vibrantly colored, mouth-watering, nutrient-rich infusions of pulverized fruits and veggies to gulp on the go for an instant healthy boost of energy. Simply swig 16 ounces of juice, and bam—you've gulped at least half of your daily nine doses of fruits and vegetables. Better health, in liquid form.

This isn't your run-of-the-mill juicing guide, though. It's packed with everything from the health benefits of cold pressing produce compared to other methods of juicing to the best ingredients to put in your juice. It includes down-to-earth and accessible explanations of crucial topics like the science behind juicing and cleansing, sound recommendations and practical advice on diet and safe juice cleansing habits, and tips and schedules that make juicing affordable and manageable no matter how busy you are.

But juice doesn't always have to be part of a challenging cleanse—it can simply be lunch that day. So for the more casual juicer, there are user-friendly tips to help personalize your cold pressing to your needs.

For those new to juicing and cleanses, there are answers to FAQs, like when you can and when you absolutely should not make juice your main dietary ingredient, the best time to juice and cleanse, and what to do when you spill a blueberry-based juice on your white shirt 30 minutes before you're due to meet with your boss. For the thrifty, there are suggestions on how to use the leftover pulp and get the most liquid bang for your produce buck. And for everyone, there are pages of tasty recipes, including variations to satisfy every craving and occasion.

Keep in mind though, that the information in this book is a useful resource, but talk to someone with an MD or RD (Registered Dietician) after their name before making long-term adjustments to your diet. While juicing is essentially a healthy choice for most diets, it could have potential harmful food-medication interactions and be harmful for diabetics, people undergoing chemotherapy, anyone who has been diagnosed with kidney disease, heart disease, hypertension or nutritional deficiencies. Now back to our regularly scheduled program.

Getting juiced has never been easier.

SECTION I
Cold Press Juicing

CHAPTER ONE
THE SKINNY

Fact: You're not eating enough vegetables and fruit. It doesn't matter if you're working up a daily sweat trying to add more crops to your diet. You could be doing everything from throwing bushels of blueberries into your morning cereal to turning your grab-a-cheese-pizza-on-the-way-home into a veritable salad bar buffet of toppings; chances are that you, like more than two-thirds of adults, aren't hitting the USDA target of nine servings of produce every day (translation: four half-cup servings of fruit and five half-cup servings of vegetables). These are not grandiose goals here. Many nutrition experts would argue that nine servings a day of fruits and vegetables is the bare minimum.

What you're missing out on could make all the difference between fizzling and sizzling health-wise. It seems we really are what we eat. Diets stuffed with fruits and vegetables not only have a heavy impact on weight management, they also reduce risk on some of the leading causes of death. According to studies from Johns Hopkins University, all it takes is one apple a day—or a peach or 10 baby carrots or a half-cup of whipped rutabaga—to lower heart disease risk by 20 percent. The Harvard School of Public Health prescribes a high dose of vegetables and fruits to help lower blood pressure, reduce the risk of cardiac disease and stroke, prevent some types of cancer, lessen the risk of eye and digestive problems, and help to lower blood sugar (the last of which, in turn, will help keep appetite in check).

In nutritional terms, vegetables especially, but also fruits, are pretty near the perfect food: low in fat and loaded with a myriad of important vitamins, minerals and antioxidants that fight all kinds of illnesses. As a study published in the *American Journal of Epidemiology* concludes, those daily nine servings, especially when eaten raw, will reduce your risk of death by as much as 10 percent and, for every extra three helpings, drop risk by another 6 percent. And, under the "It's Not Fair" heading, the benefits are even higher for those still struggling with their New Year's resolutions: When they pile on the produce, drinkers can soak up to a 40 percent mortality reduction, the obese weigh in with a 20 percent mortality reduction and there's even some evidence that smokers may also inhale some benefits. Researchers conjecture that these higher rewards may be due to antioxidants strutting their stuff which, in turn, takes the edge off the oxidative stress caused by many of these bad habits.

So the big debate isn't whether you need more fruit and vegetables in your life—you do. The question is, how you are going to get those vegetables and fruit into your body?

Hello, juice! Granted, eating vegetables in their whole form is usually the best answer. However, chomping through half of a grapefruit, a half-cup of strawberries, an apple, a banana, a cup of spinach, a half-cup of carrots, a half-cup of red peppers, a handful of asparagus stalks and a half-cup of green beans (for example) every single day can seem like the definition of impossible unless you're part groundhog. But with juice, you're literally squeezing a couple of pounds of vitamin-, mineral- and antioxidant-rich produce into a glass, which is going to be both easier and tastier to chug down.

Plus, these drinks, especially when homemade, are automatically low in the ingredients blacklisted by doctors and nutritionists. These include fats, processed sugars, artificial anything and salt. While the jury is still out on whether your body can absorb the nutrients more easily in liquid form or if there's any advantage in giving your digestive system a break from working on fiber, there is sound evidence that drinking juice delivers the goodness, and most nutrient-dense part of the food, in a concentrated form. A US Department Agriculture study found that 90 percent of the antioxidant activity, especially cancer-fighting carotenoids (which are found in carrots, spinach, apricots, tomatoes and red bell peppers, to name a few), is in the juice rather than the fiber. The *American Journal of Medicine* concluded in a study that people who quaffed 3+ servings per week of juices high in polyphenols (antioxidants found in purple grape, grapefruit, cranberry and apple juice) had a 76 percent lower risk of developing Alzheimer's disease.

The fact that the fruits and vegetables are eaten raw means that in some cases, you ingest even more of those super nutrients (see "Raw or Cooked?" on page 49 to determine when you need to turn up the heat). In short, even the most expensive vitamin pill can't begin to match the nutritional complexity of a fresh juice.

NOT YOUR BOTTLED BRAND

This juice isn't your morning gulp of Florida fresh. This juice is also a verb— juicing is the process of extracting juices from fresh fruits and vegetables using machines specifically designed to (depending on the style) either pulverize, crush or blend the produce to make a fresh and unpasteurized liquid that contains most of the vitamins, minerals and plant chemicals (phytonutrients) found in the whole fruit.

One reason juice has become a must-have for all that is good for you is that these machines are now available for home use. And although it sometimes seems like you can't throw an avocado pit these days without hitting a juice bar or a store stocked with every kind of juice from acai to zesty beet, it turns out that it pays to play Martha Stewart and juice it yourself.

While the fare at juice bars is more like homemade, it comes with the kind of sticker price usually associated with top-shelf cocktails because you're not only paying for the produce, you're subsidizing the bar's commercial version of the appliance, their real estate lease, the salaries of the workers, the monthly utility fees, the store's pet mascot and so on. In short, when it comes to juicing, there really is no place like home.

Sure, an at-home juicing machine can also be pricey and cost as much as a high-end media system (some retail for—gasp—over $10,000). But buying a juicer is like purchasing a home—you're investing for the long-term. Grabbing your juice on the hoof can run anywhere between $2 in a supermarket to $8 from a juice bar. Suddenly, going on a bender and laying out a couple of Benjamins for your own machine makes sense.

The other problem with bottled brands is that they don't always live up to their healthy hype. Juice needs to be as fresh as a just-opened bag of potato chips if you want to harvest all those five-syllable benefits like phytonutrients and antioxidants. In juice-years, anything over a day old already qualifies your drink for an AARP card. Even if your store-bought juice was made and delivered before the sun rose, it would still be older than it appears to be because it's been pasteurized so it can age with grace. In addition, it most likely has additives to keep it looking young and vibrant, and, possibly, sugar to give it a sweeter disposition. Roll up your sleeves and do the juicing yourself and you decide exactly what goes in to make an on-the-spot health drink.

This is where cold pressing really goes to the top of the class. Rather than grinding and pulverizing the veggies and fruit, which can oxidize and degrade the nutrients, this kind of no-blade juicing process slow presses and squeezes the liquid out of the produce. This means less contact with oxygen or heat, less pulp and more liquid. The result is an easily digestible, minimally processed, thicker drink filled with healthy ingredients (see "Tool Talk" on page 36 for more on the different juicing machines).

If, like My Little Pony's Rarity, you're thinking green isn't your color, know that those cold press drinks are as varied, fresh, colorful and flavorful as a Mardi Gras parade. Sure, there are supergreen juices for dense doses of nutrients, but there are also fruity juices for quick, sweet jolts, nutty milk juices for a powerful protein punch, rooty vegetables with an earthy, Birkenstock undertone, blended juices DIY-designed for whatever ails you, juices that contain hemp, chlorophyll, sprouts, spirulina and/or chia seeds to supersize your antioxidant consumption, juices that offset radio-poisoning (at least, if you're Iron Man Tony Stark; for the rest of us mere mortals, the only counteraction benefit we might reap is that the motor of some juicers will drown out bad seventies rock stations), juices that taste like salad, juices that taste like candy, juices that taste like they were conceived by the Swamp Thing and juices that somehow taste like all three and are still delish.

MODERATION MATTERS

Still, it's not quite as simple as "knock back a juice, get healthy." While juicing can offer a low-fat, nutrient-rich shot of energy, like all things dietary, the benefits are reaped when it's done in moderation as opposed to as a long-term substitute for real food. Unlike smoothies or blending, juicing squeezes out fiber. However, the Harvard School of Public Health recommends that in order to keep our poop pipes running smoothly, our tummies full, our waistlines trim, our sugar levels steady and our risk of heart disease, colon cancer, high cholesterol and diabetes low, we need to put away 14 grams of fiber for every 1,000 calories of food we eat each day (for the mathematically challenged, that adds up to 28 grams for most women and 38 grams for most men). So you either need to supplement your juices with some fiber-loaded foods or work some of the pulp back into your menu (see page 186 for more info on bulking up your pulp use, or see Chapter Three for squeezing the most goodness out of your ingredients).

Another potential dietary hazard to keep an eye out for—and one more reason to home-juice—is making sure that your juice cup does not runneth over with sugar. Juice doesn't have to be liquid candy. You can spike it with spices or lemon juice or sweeten it with a touch of sugar, but if you don't keep the drink mainly green, you'll just be drinking some Hawaiian Punch tarted up with veggies. Just memorize this ratio: 4:1. Or, if your mind leans numerically this way, 80:20 percent. This means that for every serving of fruit, you should try to take the sweet edge off with a minimum of four servings of leafy or cruciferous vegetables. (Vegetables like beets and carrots fall into a sweet, starchy black hole and should therefore not always have the star position in your juice.) You can figure out the measurements (do your calculations before you juice) with the "What Counts?" table (page 70), but don't worry about getting it exactly right. This is a rule of thumb rather than an exact formula. After all, an orange is going to produce a lot more juice than a bunch of Romaine lettuce.

Yes, you want to make your juice taste good—but with green veggies. If you throw in too many apples, grapes or bananas, it's like drinking a cup of sugar. Even 100 percent fruit juice with no natural sweeteners added can have as much sugar and as many calories as soda (or, in the case of 100 percent grape juice, as much as 50 percent more sugar; "How Sweet It Is" on page 19 breaks down the sugar content of your favorite fruits and vegetables). Yup, you read right. In a study published in the *Lancet Diabetes & Endocrinology*, researchers determined that one cup of apple juice contains 110 calories and a jaw-dropping 26 grams of sugar, which is almost the same as what you'd find in the same-size serving of cola.

Fruit is naturally jam-packed with fructose, which is essentially the molecule that makes sugar sweet (see "Sweet Science" on page 18 for a simple breakdown on the different types of sugars and how your body absorbs them). On a good day, the body gets the right amount of fructose (about 15 grams, unless you have hyperuricemia or high uric acid levels). It converts this fructose to glycogen (liver starch) as a storehouse for ready energy. This can then be fished out of your liver if your body needs glucose in the future—for instance, if you've depleted your ready stock from a heavy-duty workout or you're starving (meaning you've skipped more than a few meals—getting hungry in the slump between lunch and dinner doesn't count). So that's how it should work.

But more commonly, we feed our bodies too much fructose—and it's hard not to since it's in practically everything from agave syrup to tortilla chips to chocolate bars to raw pistachio nuts. A National Institutes of Health (NIH) study determined that the average American diet weighs in at 37+ grams of fructose daily. The problem is, too much fructose and our digestive system—specifically the liver—becomes overwhelmed and unable to process it fast enough for the body to use as sugar.

Sure, the sugar from that soda is processed and the sugar from produce is Mama Nature's best. But it actually makes no difference if the fructose is from too much fruit or too much junk food—all fructose works the same in the body. Like that out-of-control conveyor belt from the classic *I Love Lucy* candy factory episode, the liver goes haywire and starts making fats from the fructose and sending them into the bloodstream as triglycerides (a type of fat or lipid in your blood and an important measure of heart health). This can have a three-pronged effect: 1) substantially increased risk of heart disease, high cholesterol, liver disease, some cancers and gout; 2) since the fructose does an end run around the body's appetite signal system, the mind doesn't register that it's full, which leads to overeating and weight gain; and 3) screaming panic headlines tarring fruit juice as a major cause for type 2 diabetes risk (British

Medical Association) and worse for you than a Krispy Kreme donut (Credit Suisse Research Institute).

However, there's no danger in juicing and there are a load of benefits as long as you stick to the 4:1 ratio. Giving the vegetables the starring role and the fruit a bit part in your juice means you'll also soften some of the stronger flavors of those mega-healthy greens. By throwing in the odd apple or orange as a sweetener, you create a glass of healthy goodness any nutritionist would want to drink. In this mix, homemade juice truly becomes the ultimate convenience food: You don't even have to chew, or, in many cases, cook. You just have it your way.

Scan the table on the following page to find out the total sugar profile (sucrose, glucose and fructose) of some common vegetable and fruit cold pressed juice ingredients in flavor combos that will make your taste buds dance.

SWEET SCIENCE

Sugar has become the bogeyman of nutrition. It makes us fat. It's toxic. It causes our skin to break out and our teeth to decay. It makes us go on spending sprees. It's actually an E.T. and has a master plan to take over the world. We need to eliminate it from our diets, our lives, the planet.

Yes, sugar lends its weight to obesity, heart disease, diabetes and a slew of other health conditions and, yes, sugar is big agribusiness (the US is one of the world's largest producers of sugar crops), and yes, it can even make us act irrationally (a sugar high has successfully been used to show diminished mental capacity as part of a manslaughter defense). But the truth, plain and simple, is our bodies run on sugar. Here's how it works in 10 easy-to-digest sound bites:

1. Whether a carbohydrate is sweet (like table sugar or in fruit) or not (as in bread or vegetables), all carbs can be broken down in the body into sugar.

2. If it ends in "ose," it's a sugar.

How Sweet It Is

Veggie 1	Veggie 2	Veggie 3	Fruit	Little Something Extra	Total Sugar (grams)
2 cups cabbage (4.4g)	1 cup fennel (.0g)	1 cup cucumber with peel (2g)	1 cup pear with peel (14g)	3 sprigs cilantro (.0g)	20.4g
2 cups spinach (.2g)	1 cup beets (9g)	1 cup carrots with peel (5g)	1 cup oranges (17g)	1 sprig rosemary (.0g)	31.2g
2 cups kale (.0g)	1 cup red cabbage (3g)	1 cup cucumber with peel (2g)	1 cup blueberries (15g)	2 sprigs lavender (.0g)	20.0g
2 cups Romaine lettuce (2g)	2 cups broccoli (3.2g)	1 inch ginger (.2g)	1 cup apple with peel (13g)	2 sprigs mint (.0g)	18.4 g
2 cups Swiss chard (.8g)	1 cup beets (9g)	1 cup red cabbage (3g)	1 cup apple with peel (13g)	1 tablespoon spirulina (.25g)	26.05g
2 cups bok choy (1.6g)	1 cup watercress (.1g)	1 cup cucumber with peel (2g)	1 cup mango (24g)	½ cup basil (.0g)	27.7g
2 cups kale (.0g)	1 cup celery (2g)	1 cup cucumber with peel (2g)	1 ounce dark chocolate 70–85% cacao solids (7g)	dash black pepper (.0g)	11.0g
2 cups spinach (.2g)	1 cup cabbage (4.4g)	1 cup beets (9g)	1 cup orange (17g)	2 tablespoons cacao powder (.0g)	30.6g
2 cups spinach (.2g)	1 cup tomatoes (3.2g)	1 cup zucchini (2g)	1 cup apple with peel (13g)	1 small chipotle pepper (.0g)	18.4g
2 cups Swiss chard (.8g)	1 cup cabbage (4.4g)	1 lime (1g)	1 cup grapes (15g)	1 tablespoon honey (17g)	38.2g

3. There are two main kinds of sugar: monosaccharides, or simple sugars, and disaccharides, or complex sugars (essentially the unromantic scientific term describing when two monosaccharides get hitched).

4. Most foods, including fruits, vegetables, dairy products and grains, contain some monosaccharides. Meats and oils are among the few foods that don't contain any sugar.

5. There are three types of monosaccharides:

   ○ Glucose: The most common of the monosaccharides, this is the sugar our bodies want to use for energy.

   ○ Fructose: Most commonly found in fruit, this sugar also occurs naturally in honey and agave syrup.

   ○ Galactose: This is mostly only in milk.

6. Mother Nature likes symmetry so there are also three types of disaccharides:

   ○ Sucrose: Glucose + Fructose (think table sugar)

   ○ Maltose: Glucose + Glucose (aka malt sugar)

   ○ Lactose: Glucose + Galactose (milk sugar by any other name)

7. Ideally, when you eat any of these sugars, your body will break them down into glucose (the body's number one go-to for energy) fairly rapidly. Monosaccharide is absorbed right into the bloodstream (fructose is broken down in the liver first) while disaccharide is first digested so enzymes split them up into their monosaccharide components, after which the body handles it as if you ate the single sugar directly.

8. Unfortunately, chances are that your body already has more than enough sugar to burn as energy, thank you very much, so it ends up converting the sugars to be stored in your fat cells. This causes your pancreas to do a sugar dance and release a hormone called insulin, whose job it is to deal with all of that excess glucose by parking it in the liver and muscles as glycogen and in the fat cells as triglycerides. The more sugar in the bloodstream, the more insulin is released, which ultimately results in our blood sugar dropping below normal levels. This, ironically, makes us crave more sugar.

9. The more sugar you eat, the higher the sugar spike, the more insulin is released and the more likely it is for your glucose to go directly to fat storage without stopping as an energy source first.

10. The sweet news is that vegetables and, in moderation, fruit are a healthy source of monosaccharides, so they actually help keep appetite (and blood sugar) in check.

DECODING THE LABELS

Your cheat sheet to learning the lingo for buying produce, juice and sweeteners—no nutrition degree required:

MADE FROM CONCENTRATE: Make sure the label also includes "100 percent fruit juice with no added sugar." In a perfect world, concentrating juice removes all water from the juice, end of story. Nothing else is added or removed. This is usually accomplished by using heat to evaporate the water; what remains are the sugars and flavonoids that give the juice its flavor. Once the juice is in concentrated form, it can be frozen and stored for extended periods of time. This would all be fine and good except for one thing: the degree of Brix in the concentrate. A degree of Brix is a unit of measurement for sugar dissolved in water; 1 degree of Brix is equivalent to 1 gram of sugar dissolved in 100 ml of water. So 30 degrees Brix is going to equal 30 grams of sugar per 100 ml of water, and so on. In order for a juice to be considered 100 percent juice, it either has to be not-from-concentrate or from concentrate but has the identical Brix value of its not from concentrate cousin and no additional ingredients—just concentrated juice and water. Here's where it gets tricky: When the concentrated juice is reconstituted, water—and only water—should be added until the juice reaches its preconcentrated Brix level. But sometimes, it's difficult to achieve nature's perfect sugar:water ratio. So the process begins to resemble a *MythBusters* moment—add a little sugar to up the Brix level, add some water because too much sugar was added, and so on. If this happens, the drink cannot be labeled 100 percent juice.

100 PERCENT JUICE: Finally, juice and nothing but juice. Actually, not quite. Yes, juice labeled 100 percent will contain a single or a blend of different fruit and/

or vegetable juice that is either squeezed directly from the produce or made from concentrated juice (see "Made from Concentrate" on the previous page). Yes, it has no added sugars, sweeteners, colors or additives. But it might be supplemented with vitamins and or minerals (most commonly, the bone-building nutrients calcium and vitamin D, which are more likely to be found in dairy foods—go figure). Also, while the "100 percent juice" label means that everything in the bottle came from a fruit or vegetable, it may not necessarily be the fruit or vegetable you think you're gulping. To save money, companies dilute more expensive produce like pomegranate and cranberry with cheaper juices like white grape, apple or pear. The finished product is still 100 percent fruit juice, but it may not necessarily be juice from the fruit you were expecting.

JUICE COCKTAIL, JUICE DRINK AND JUICE-FLAVORED BEVERAGE: Eye opener—a box of fruit-sweetened cereal might contain more actual fruit than these drinks! Their real juice content can range anywhere from 10 percent to 99.9 percent of the drink (although the numbers usually hover somewhere between 10 percent to 50 percent). The main ingredients are usually water and some type of sugar (see "AKA Sugar" on page 26), plus added sweeteners, flavors and other additives.

FRUIT-FLAVORED DRINKS: Often, no fruits were harmed in the making of these drinks. Usually a brew of lab-concocted sweeteners and flavorings splice fruity flavors with a fortification of vitamins and minerals to make them look nutritious; these drinks have none of the antioxidants and phytochemicals found in actual fruit and vegetable juices.

"MADE WITH REAL FRUIT" OR "CONTAINS REAL FRUIT JUICE": One grape or one drop of orange juice can make this claim accurate. However, a quick look at the ingredients list will show you what you need to know. Ingredients are listed from the most to least abundant on the ingredients list. This pecking order also applies to 100 percent juice, so if your Pomegranate Blend boasts apple juice as the first ingredient and pomegranate as the last, you're drinking much less pomegranate juice and mostly very expensive apple juice.

NOT FROM CONCENTRATE: Don't take off your reading glasses just yet. The drink might still have added flavors, even if it is labeled 100 percent fruit juice. For instance, storage makes the juice lose its flavor so the solution the food scientists came up with is to add lab-produced essence to give the juice its original tang. There are no requirements for companies to label that the juice has been "re-flavored."

ORGANIC: This is the only label that delivers the full grocery cart of nutritional goods (see "Organic or Conventional?" on page 48 for when you can skip this label). For a food to bear the USDA Organic symbol, it must meet strict criteria, including having no synthetic ingredients, petroleum-based fertilizers, synthetic pesticides or anything that's been genetically modified.

ALL NATURAL/NATURAL: Your red flag to scan the ingredients label—the FDA requires only that these foods contain no added color, artificial flavors or synthetic substances. So "natural" foods can still contain up to 90 percent chemically processed ingredients, such as high fructose corn syrup (some companies argue that since it comes from corn, it's healthy), alkalized cocoa, partially hydrogenated soybean oil, vanillin and maltodextrin. Even 100 percent natural isn't necessarily 100 percent synthetic free—Naked Juice (owned by PepsiCo) settled a lawsuit in 2013 because they claimed their juices were 100 percent all natural but really contained things like Fibersol-2 (a proprietary synthetic digestion-resistant fiber produced by Archer Daniels Midland and developed by a Japanese chemical company—yum), fructooligosaccharides (it's easier to say that it's a synthetic fiber and sweetener) and Inulin (an artificial and invisible fiber added to foods to artificially increase fiber content).

NATURAL FLAVORS: This means as much as a blind date saying "I'll call you in the morning" in ingredient-labeling terms. In officialese, natural flavors could be "the essential oil, oleoresin, essence or extractive, protein hydrolysate, distillate, or any product of roasting, heating or enzymolysis, which contains the flavoring constituents derived from a spice, fruit or fruit juice, vegetable or vegetable juice, edible yeast, herb, bark, bud, root, leaf or similar plant material, meat, seafood, poultry, eggs, dairy products, or fermentation products thereof, whose significant function in food is flavoring rather than nutritional" (source: US Food and Drug Administration Code of Federal Regulations, Title 21). In real speak, it must derive from real food. In realest speak, your juice could legally include beaver butt (aka castoreum, which is an extraction of the dried glands and secretions from a beaver's rear end, used to create, most often, a vanilla flavor). One more thing: Both artificial and natural flavors are made by "flavorists" in a laboratory by blending either "natural" chemicals or "synthetic" chemicals to create flavorings. By the time they're finished, processing will have distilled these "natural" flavorings from anything recognizable as the original source (which may be a good thing if it's castoreum).

ADDED VITAMINS OR MINERALS: Like an athlete on steroids, companies pump nutrients into drinks and food to make them sound healthier. A carton of OJ has so many added vitamins that its container looks like an ABC book. Some bottles of juice claim to help with weight loss and reduce risk of heart attack and stroke. It sounds good, but the evidence shows that these "functional foods" may also contain a list of unhealthy ingredients like sugar and fat and in no way equate to consuming real foods that naturally contain these nutritional benefits.

COLORS AND DYES: Creepy crawlies, anyone? Cochineal and carmine, made from the bodies of a scaly female insect, are used to add those vibrant hues to foods like grapefruit juice, lemonade and applesauce. Lab-made FD&C Green No. 3 and Fast Green FCF might give vegetable juice a faux healthy hue. These shades are chemically injected into food to make them resemble the pleasing eat-me-now colors that nature produces naturally—like reds, oranges and yellows.

NO PRESERVATIVES: They might not have been treated with ingredients that sound like they belong in a chemistry set (citric acid, sulfur dioxide, ascorbic acid, propionic acid, nitrates and nitrites, sodium bisulfite, sulfites and even formaldehyde are all used as food preservatives to slow or prevent spoilage, discoloration, flavor loss, bacterial growth, mold or microbial growth and texture loss). But even food with a "No Preservatives" shout-out may have been blasted with irradiation to help keep it from spoiling—and this includes fresh fruit and vegetables, seeds for sprouting and herbs and spices (in other words, the ingredients of a glass of juice). But before you take the 100 percent preservative-free vow, know that if the commercial drink you buy truly lives up to this label, it may then be laced with mold. Researchers at Indiana State University uncovered five species of the fungus in one popular drink (named for a Mediterranean holiday destination) because its no preservative maxim meant that when the packaging was damaged, air seeped in which, in turn, encouraged the fungus to grow.

PASTEURIZATION: This is the process of heating food, usually a liquid, to kill pathogens and prevent spoilage. While there's a warehouse of papers debating whether pasteurization is harmful, there's no hard data showing exactly what side effects it has on the nutritional value of juice. While it's good that harmful pathogens are destroyed through pasteurization, it's also possible that beneficial enzymes and proteins are being destroyed in the process.

GMOS OR GENETICALLY MODIFIED ORGANISMS: Although not required to be labeled as such, these are Frankenstein plants or animals that have had DNA added to their genes from different species of living organisms, bacteria or viruses to get desired traits such as resistance to disease or tolerance of pesticides. Although present in up to 70 percent of foods on US supermarket shelves, according to the Center for Food Safety, the good news is that the only GM produce you're likely to find in the produce aisles is the Hawaiian papaya, a small amount of zucchini and squash, and some sweet corn.

IRRADIATED: An evil twin of GMOs, the method of treating food with irradiation was first approved by the FDA in 1963 to control insects in wheat and flour. Food (mostly spices and a little bit of meat and poultry) is passed through irradiation (as opposed to heated, which is the energy source in pasteurization) to kill pathogens. It doesn't make the food radioactive any more than passing X-rays through your body makes you radioactive; it just causes changes in the food. While those changes result in the mass destruction of any E. coli or salmonella that might be present in food, the concern is that they also destroy nutrients that are definitely part of the food's DNA. But you don't get to decide if you want to skip food that has been irradiated because there are no label laws regarding it.

CITRIC ACID: This is included as a standalone because so many juices use it to extend the shelf life of their product. You would think with a name that includes "citric," a lemon, orange, lime or grapefruit must have been involved in the making of this preservative. Think again. More likely, it was made from GMO corn and sugar beets. (Isn't science amazing?)

GREEN LABELS: Literally, labels colored green. A sneaky marketing tool to lull you into thinking the food is healthier, according to research published in the journal *Health Communication*.

SERVING SIZE: A small bottle of juice may actually contain four portions; to make a product look low in fat or calories, manufacturers base the nutritional content on small, often unrealistic, serving sizes (this might change as new label laws are being hammered out).

CORN SUGAR: This is not high fructose corn syrup. Nor does it contain even a droplet of fructose. But that is only because corn sugar is what corn syrup in all its guises is made from. However, it's an excess of sugar that is bad for us. It just turns out that corn syrup, high fructose or not, is one of the most common sweeteners in processed food—even in items you wouldn't expect it to show up in, like whole wheat bread, honey roasted peanuts, frozen pizza and tonic water. So the real watchword to be on the lookout for is "sugar" or its 30 aliases (see "AKA Sugar," below).

SUGAR-FREE: Shock, horror, gasp! Foods labeled "sugar-free" may not actually be 100 percent sugar-free. These products often contain sugar alcohols, which are lower in calories (roughly 2 calories per gram, compared to 4 per gram for sugar), but they still contain calories and carbohydrates from other sources.

NO SUGAR ADDED: Fruits and vegetables naturally contain sugar, so although these products may not have added sugar, they still may contain natural sugars.

LIGHTLY SWEETENED: A marketer's made-up term that is the verbal equivalent of "I only cheated a little." In other words, it means nothing.

"FAT FREE": This label is often stamped on 100 percent juices—truthful, but duh!

AKA SUGAR

Unlike a rose, a tablespoon of sugar is not a tablespoon of sugar is not... etc. Refined sugars have gone through some sort of processing to be produced and may also include chemicals (it's not uncommon for refined sugars to sweeten their look and shelf life with small amounts of carbon dioxide, phosphoric acid or calcium hydroxide). But unrefined sugars don't get an automatic sweet pass. The sour truth is that overindulging in even the few sugars that retain some nutrients after production (such as blackstrap molasses and maple syrup) can potentially lead to a slew of health conditions (a higher risk of obesity, high blood pressure, dementia, type 2 diabetes, dyslipidemia—a bad assortment of blood fats—cirrhosis of the liver and cardiovascular disease are among the health concerns of eating or drinking too much of any kind of sugar).

Unfortunately, it's not easy to identify what is sweetening your drink. Companies have started to disguise the sugar in their beverages by using different names. Here are 30 (!) of the most popular pseudonyms for sugar:

Agave nectar

Barley malt

Blackstrap molasses

Brown palm sugar

Brown sugar (common light and dark)

Cane crystals

Cane sugar

Corn sweetener

Corn syrup

Crystalline fructose

Date sugar

Dextrose

Evaporated cane juice

Fructose

Fruit juice concentrates

Fruit sugar

Glucose

High fructose corn syrup

Honey

Invert sugar

Lactose

Malt syrup

Maltose

Maple syrup

Palm sugar

Raw sugar

Sucanat

Sucrose

Syrup

Turbinado sugar

IN THE JUICE

Turns out a liquid lunch can actually be good for you. Here are ten reasons why you should start getting juiced:

1. You'll impress your doctor because unlike two-thirds of Americans, you really will be hitting—and probably exceeding—your daily fruit and veggie quotient. Better yet, you'll be doing it without forcing your taste buds into submission. Unlike non-alcoholic beer, decaffeinated coffee and all those other drinks otherwise known as "If It Tastes Bland, It Must Be Good for You," a freshly made juice is actually delicious.

2. Your doctor may look up to you, literally. Greens such as kale, collards and broccoli are high in the nutrients calcium and magnesium (juicing is like making a multipurpose vitamin!), both of which are crucial for a strong, healthy skeleton.

3. You'll remember to go to your doctor. An NIH study found that a diet high in fruit and vegetables boosts brain power and, in some cases, wards off dementia and cognitive decline.

4. You won't sleep through your doctor's appointment. You may not get the sudden super strength and muscle mass of Popeye, but research from the National Heart, Lung, and Blood Institute found that leafy vegetables like kale and spinach are packed with iron that boosts red blood circulation, making you feel more energetic, alert and able to concentrate. Greek studies of athletes found that drinking tomato juice results in quicker levels of muscle recovery after going for the burn.

5. Actually, you probably won't really need to go to the doctor. Numerous studies have determined that getting your full prescription of produce can protect your body from deadly chronic conditions such as heart disease, diabetes and cancer.

6. You won't even need to go away on vacation. Fresh juice is rich in nutrients like vitamin C and magnesium, which have a mellowing effect, helping your body better combat the effects of the stress hormone cortisol and improving the quality of your sleep so that you feel as rested as you would after a week away.

7. But you'll look like you've been on a beach vacay. Research from the University of Nottingham suggests eating a healthy diet rich in fruit and vegetables gives you a more healthy golden glow than the sun.

8. You'll also become more adventurous without ever leaving your house—or even, once you've pressed, your couch. Juicing encourages you to eat a lot of vegetables and fruit you never thought you would. Frankly, chances are low you were going to sit down on a daily basis to a stack of kale and collard greens, a bucket of wheat grass, a cup of chlorophyll, a passel of different kinds of veggies and fruit like blood oranges, bull beets, dino kale and white

carrots, to name a few. There are thought to be over 2,000 different known varieties of fruits and vegetables—that's a lot of juice to try.

9. You'll have earned your cleansing badge. Cleansing is simply shorthand in our fast and busy times for "liquid fasting." These cleanses can be as intense or as low-key as you want (see Chapter Four for the nitty gritty on cleansing and Chapter Five for specific cleanse plans). Most people cleanse for anywhere from a 24-hour rinse to a full, seven-day cycle (or more, though a liquids-only diet isn't a healthy choice beyond one week unless you're adding protein and fiber to the mix). But cleansing is really more about shifting yourself into a healthier state of mind and body than counting the axis rotations of the earth. So if unhealthy foods are regularly eating away your daily diet, try switching a fresh juice for one of your usual alcohol, soda or junk food servings every day. Increase on an hourly/daily/weekly/whatever-works-for-you basis until you've completely drunk your way out of your bad habits. Ergo, you're now cleansed.

10. You'll live forever. Or at least a very, very, very long time. Studies done by the Minerva Institute for Medical Research show that nutrients often found in fresh juice, such as resveratrol, keep cells from prematurely dying, increasing longevity and keeping you healthy to boot.

CHAPTER TWO
SETTING UP YOUR HOME JUICE BAR

In a taste smackdown, homemade juice is not necessarily always going to win out over store-bought juice. Blended with over 20 different ingredients ranging from cacao nibs, Bosc pear, shiso leaves, blood orange marmalade, echinacea, chlorella, barley grass, Jerusalem artichoke, Nova Scotia dulse, kiwi puree and dried Black Mission figs, as well as the requisite kale and spinach, a sip of some commercial juices merit their own sommelier.

But it turns out that despite this, you will like them apples—and kale, mango, ginger, chia seeds, lime and parsley—just fine, thank you very much. While you may not have access to the kind of ingredients that might show up in the mystery basket on *Chopped*, what you do have in your produce basket when juicing at home is hands-on control. Not only do you not know what the vegetable to fruit ratio is when you buy your juice over the counter, you might also lose out on freshness, quality, rawness and purity because you don't always have the skinny on the additives, sugar levels, age and organic label of the produce being blended to give off-the-shelf potions that drink-me-now hue and taste. So setting up your own home juice bar is always going to be the healthier option.

It's also the most convenient option for a busy life. Having your own juicer may mean laying out some serious bucks, but it's like having your very own "reset" button in that you can cold press whenever you need to overhaul your diet (like every Monday), making it a much more useful appliance than that corn kernel remover you thought you just had to have.

But it turns out that how your juicer whips up your ingredients impacts just how much nutrition makes its way into your glass. Like potatoes and tomatoes, juicers may belong to the same (appliance) family, but their hardware DNA will differ. There are essentially two categories of juicers—centrifugal and masticating (see "The Backups" on page 34 for a roundup of other types of juicers). The difference has to do with the way the machines extract and separate the juice from the pulp. A description of the way they work can read like a rating from a dating site: cheap and fast (centrifugal), slow and strong (masticating) and high-maintenance (the backups).

HARDCORE JUICERS VS. EVERYONE ELSE

Hardcore Juicers or HJs (see "How can I become a Hardcore Juicer?" in Chapter Seven) swear that you absolutely must have the following five appliances to liquefy your produce properly:

1. A high-speed blender to pre-pulverize soft, pulpy fruits like blueberries, peaches and strawberries that are slow to juice and may clog up the mesh screen in a masticating juicer;

2. A citrus juicer (you'll get more juice and won't have to peel the fruit as you might with some of the other juicers);

3. A mini food processor/grinder for seeds and nuts;

4. A wheatgrass juicer;

5. At least one kind (but preferably all three different types) of juicer.

If you are like everyone else—that is, you indulge in (vegan) chocolate too often, don't own yoga pants (unless your PJs count), would just as soon ask the dentist to extract your teeth to keep you from eating too much as you would have a voluntary colonic procedure, and don't go by the name Dusk, Rainbow or Blue—can happily get by juicing with just one machine.

CHOOSING YOUR MACHINE

Cheap and fast, the centrifugal juicer is the darling of juicer infomercials. They use blades, a grater or a shredder disc to grind your ingredients before spinning them at around 35,000 revolutions per minute, or RPM (think wet clothes in the laundry spin cycle). The force pushes the juice through a strainer basket with the pulp and separates the pulp into a separate compartment.

At first glance, these juicers seem the perfect match for most lifestyles and budgets. They often have a wide feed chute and small blades so they can slice and dice whole, firm produce like carrots, beets and apples quicker than a chef at Benihana—so less prep work for you. However, while centrifugal juicers may win the race to your glass, they lose on nutrition. It turns out that that big mouth and those tiny sharp teeth can't handle the healthier produce like leafy greens and wheatgrass. Plus, the high speed and heat generated from the blades may compromise the living nutrients and enzymes found in whole fruit and vegetables, so the juice—a pale, foamy liquid that resembles something only a cow could love—needs to be drunk immediately after it's extracted from the juicer. The juicers themselves also tend to be noisy and spit, so the time you save cutting produce will probably be used cleaning juice splatters from your ceiling.

Slow and strong, like the hero of a Jane Austen novel, cold press juicers, aka masticating or single-gear juicers, are the kind most of the juice bars use. Unlike centrifugals and most other juicers, these brawny machines can take on just about any ingredient, from amaranth, burdock and cabbage to yams, xigua (Chinese watermelon) and zingiber (type of ginger), as well as those leafy greens often lacking in everyday diets, and cold press them to a healthy, nutrient-rich, colorful drink.

What makes cold press juicers a healthier option than the centrifugals is their blend of versatility, thriftiness and thoroughness. Although they cost more initially, this is one of those times when, as Grandpa used to say, quality counts. Cold press machines simply can't be beat when it comes to maximum juice extraction. Instead of chewing up the produce, they work like a medieval torture device, using a wormlike gear known as an auger to grind and crush the fruits and vegetables though a screen, squeezing every last drop of juice from the meat, skin and seeds of the fruit and vegetables to the point where nothing's left but a thin, dry crisp. So your drink isn't only pulped with more fiber, it includes more juice from your produce, ounce for ounce. Although your initial outlay on a cold press juicer will be higher, you'll save money in the long run on ingredients.

Even a low-end cold press juicer will squeeze out more and thicker juice from whatever you put in it than the priciest centrifugal juicer—and the juice will have more nutrients because you won't be restricted from using divas of the vegetable world (difficult to work with but incredibly vitamin-rich), like leafy greens and wheatgrasses. Plus the slow rotations in cold press juicers (which turn between 80–120 RPM) eliminate the oxidization and heating that occurs with centrifugals (which zip around anywhere from 3,000–16,000 RPM), so the ingredients' enzymes and nutrients are preserved closest to their natural form. The visual translation: An apple juiced on a centrifugal juicer will cough up an oxidized brownish-colored separated juice while an apple juiced on a cold press machine juicer will result in brightly colored, even-colored, thicker nectar.

The machines themselves also generally last longer because they don't undergo as much wear and tear as the centrifugals with their whirring spin cycles and blades. In fact, companies generally provide longer warranties on cold press juicers as their life expectancy is much greater and parts are designed to be more durable. The lack of noisy parts also means that cold press juicers are ultra-quiet, so you won't wake up your entire household when you juice first thing in the morning and that morning juice will last about 72 hours longer without compromising its nutritional integrity.

Some cold press juicers are designed to work horizontally, a simple adjustment that transforms the machine into a multipurpose food processor that can mince, grind, chop, shave ice and make soy milk, nut butters, pasta, hummus, pesto, tomato sauce, raw applesauce, baby food and sorbet (practically the only thing these babies can't do is wash windows). The vertical versions are not quite as versatile, but they have bigger mouths so less time is needed to prepare the produce and they take up less counter space so you'll still have room for your food processor.

Practically the only frowny-face is that these juicers have narrow chutes, so you'll need to put in more prep work as the ingredients must be cut into smaller pieces to fit. But even that can be balanced out by the time you'll save cleaning up—as opposed to centrifugals, the parts on cold press juicers detach easily and can usually be thrown into the dishwasher.

THE BACKUPS

If you know a teenage girl, then you know that almost every boy band is made up of five members with very distinct personalities. The same goes for these juicers—each has some unique aspect that might appeal to a small segment of the juicing population, but none could be truly categorized as an all-around affordable performer:

1. The Bad Boy Type (think JC Chasez from *NSYNC, Donnie Wahlberg from NKOTB or Zayn Malik from One Direction): Mega Blender
You've invested in a mega blender and it's like an appliance on steroids, flexing its muscles around your kitchen. Which lulls you into thinking that it'll easily handle pureeing a few veggies and fruits into a fresh green juice. Warning: You may ultimately get the results you want, but, as is often the case with bad boys, you're going to have to work much harder for them than you would with a purpose-made juicer—more chopping, more blending and more heavy lifting to extract a juice that has fewer nutrients and more exposure to oxygen. Moral? Stay away from bad boys when it comes to juicing!

2. The Sweet and Innocent Type (think Nick Carter from Backstreet Boys [then, not now], or Niall Horan from One Direction): The Manual Leverage Presser
Full of nostalgic charm, the manual leverage presser is really a fancy name for Gram's old citrus press. It's durable (Gram's is probably still good to go), affordable and low-maintenance, but the results are bland. Sure it makes the kind of juice any Floridian would be proud of, but it takes a lot of elbow grease to coax out the results and it's limited in that the kind of juice it makes is citrus, just citrus and nothing but citrus.

3. The Class Clown (think Danny Wood from NKOTB, Joey Fatone from *NSYNC or Louis Tomlinson from One Direction): Wheatgrass Juicer

The green drinks made by dedicated wheatgrass juicers are definitely the life of the juicing party—cost-efficient, vibrant, tangy and full of life. You can go low-tech with a hand crank or upgrade to an electric version. They both essentially work the same way: cold press and squeeze, like mangle-wringing a wet cloth. Extra patience is needed with either type as they're slow and, even with the electric, some effort is needed to operate. Eventually, their one-note ingredient can wear thin and you start to yearn for some more complexity to your juices.

4. The Strong, Silent Type (think Lass Bass from *NSYNC, Jonathan Knight from NKOTB or Liam Payne from One Direction): Hydraulic Press

Capable and solid, the hydraulic press can always be depended on to produce delicious healthy juice. The press might be hand or electrically powered. The latter design is based on the Norwalk Ultimate Juicer, which is the first commercially known juicer and still around today. Pre-ground fruits and vegetable pulp is wrapped in special filtering (usually linen) cloth and squeezed between two stainless steel plates via a hydraulic pump. While the hydraulic juice press electrically tends to be high-quality, the downsides—and there are several—are these machines tend to be pricey (that Norwalk can set you back around $2,000), time consuming to use and fiddly to clean.

The advantage of the manual hydraulic press is that no electricity needed, it requires fewer parts so it's less complicated and less likely to break down, you control how fast the press goes and how long the ingredients stay compressed (you could walk away mid-press and answer the phone or work out). On the other hand, you'll need to pump up your biceps to extract enough juice to last the day.

5. The Stud (think Jordan Knight From NKOTB, Justin Timberlake from *NSYNC, Brian Littrell from Backstreet Boys or Harry Styles from One Direction): Triturating or Twin-Gear Juicer

The triturating or twin-gear juicer stands out as one sexy machine—and comes with the price tag to prove it (some run as high as $2,500). You may need to splash out even more money on a fruit attachment. These juicers are really designed for those Hardcore Juicers (page 31) who live on liquids and need a machine that can extract the highest volume of juice, fiber and nutrients (although some turn their noses up at the triturating, saying they produce smoothies rather than juice). The mechanisms turn at a tortoise speed of about 80 RPM, cold pressing foods between two interlocking gears which first shred, then squeeze produce. Like the best studs, triturators can handle everything thrown at them with street smart cool and will juice practically anything, including squashes, Brazil nuts and pine needles (seriously). But more patience is required as the small feeding chute makes feeding it challenging. Some triturators even have fancy magnetic and bio-ceramic technology to slow down the oxidation process so juice can be stored without losing out on any As, Bs or Cs.

TOOL TALK

Your cold press juicer is going to be just as integral to your daily life as any major appliance in your house, so be smart before you start shopping. It's easy to get distracted by all the bells and whistles (hands up if you've ever almost bought a car because it came with a heated seat gizmo). With so many models offering high-speed this and extra-pasta-making that, it can be head-spinning to figure out what you actually need. Is there really any difference between a juicer that costs $30 and one that costs the same as your monthly rent? After all, don't they all make juice? Well, yes and no.

The reality is if you're a beginner juicer, most cold pressers probably will do the trick. But if this is something that you're planning to do long-term, you might as well make the money plunge to find one that truly suits your needs (see "Juicers Worth Your Squeeze" on page 38 to find the best cold press juicer match for your lifestyle) because this is probably going to be a one-time purchase. Cold press juicers are like Oldsmobiles and built to last. One way to look at the cost is that it's an investment in your health—feel better now?

To avoid buyer's remorse (and your shiny expensive new toy being shoved in the back of your deepest cupboard), check off your priorities from the list of options below and use the resulting must-haves when you start comparison shopping to get the best model with the best combo of features at the best price.

$200 OR UNDER PRICE TAG: There are some more-than-decent smooth operators that won't clean out your wallet (the Bella Nutripro gets five stars for delivering the goods at an affordable price). However, there is such a thing as too good to be true. The chilly, hard truth is that most cold press juicers are going to cash out in the $300–$500 range. Really cheap models will end up costing you more in effort; for instance, anything under $50 is probably a manual cold press (so you supply the press power) and may actually end up being more expensive in the long run as they'll probably burn out more quickly and therefore need replacing.

EASY-TO-UNDERSTAND INSTRUCTIONS: Don't even look at that seductive all-stainless, automatic pulp rejection, twin-gear press system without first taking a look at the operating manual. If it makes you feel dazed and confused, like you were teleported back to your 11th grade physics class, or the directions aren't in a language you recognize (one inexpensive juicer comes with a manual in French), then this isn't your perfect appliance.

LONG CORD: If you tend to get tangled in extension cords and don't have multiple outlets in your kitchen, a short power lead could be a deal breaker.

CHUTE FEEDER SIZE: If you don't have the knife skills or the time to cut your ingredients down to size, take note of the chute's measurements. Cold pressers tend to be narrow-mouthed (usually under two inches, although some come in at three).

DISHWASHER-SAFE, REMOVABLE PIECES: If you have a dishwasher, you don't want to be hand-washing your juicer parts.

IT COMES IN A SIZE THAT'S SMALLER THAN AN ELEPHANT BUT BIGGER THAN A BREADBOX: The juicer may have to share living space with all of the other appliances on your kitchen counter or you might decide to keep it in your cupboard except when juicing (warning: this plan probably won't last longer than the first week, after which you realize that you're going to be firing up this baby too often to bother hauling it in and out all of the time). Some take up more than their share of elbow room, so shop with a tape measure and know your space limitations—this is one instance where you might not want to supersize. Also, don't be seduced by a high-end, good-looking model. Beauty is as beauty does, and while your juicer may have the sleek lines of a fancy racing car, you might be able to hand-squeeze a gallon of juice faster than it can press out a single ounce of liquid.

IT CAN BE REPAIRED LOCALLY: Cold press juicers are known for their longevity, but it may still need the odd tweaking and you don't want to apply for a passport to keep your machine running smoothly.

IT FOLLOWS THE RULE "LESS IS MORE": Fewer moving parts means faster and easier clean up. Stainless steel is the most durable and simplest material to maintain. Also look for pulp receptacles and a filter screen that are easy to remove—some need a full toolkit and a degree in mechanical engineering to extract for cleaning.

A THREE-YEAR-OLD COULD USE IT: If the functions are confusing, cumbersome or a chore, you won't use your juicer. Your machine should be easy to operate and easy to clean so the only thing dictating when you whip up a juice is your mood.

IT GIVES YOU THE FULL BOUNTY: You want a juicer that can produce the goods. You may end up saving money on the juicer but then paying—and paying—for more vegetables and fruit because your less-expensive model just doesn't have what it takes to squeeze every last drop out. A high-quality juicer will leave you with nothing but pulp dust, so what you laid out initially in equipment cost is quickly recouped in food savings.

JUICERS WORTH YOUR SQUEEZE

Maybe your plan to start cold pressing your produce is doomed from the start because you don't like chopping veggies or you hate waiting longer than a heartbeat for anything. A Harvard School of Public Health study found that people are more likely to stick with their get-healthy plan if they find the right MO for their lifestyle. The list below matches the cold press juicer to your daily needs:

YOU'RE A JUICING VIRGIN: Your juicer shouldn't have more buttons than a 747. If you're new to juicing, all you need are the basics: an on/off switch, something energy- and cost-efficient, with safety features and easy to clean. The Breville BJS600XL Fountain Crush Masticating Slow Juicer is a good-value starter machine. It makes cold press juicing as hassle-free and KISS (keep it simple, stupid) as it can get. It combines all features that a professional juicer would like and is easy enough to be used by a complete beginner. It has a "safe start" function so it gets going only once all its parts are securely locked in their respected places, an overload protection system (so no OMG overflow messes) and an easy auto-clean system (just add hot water).

YOU'D RATHER HAVE YOUR NAILS RIPPED OFF THAN ASK FOR DIRECTIONS: The Hurom HU-100 juicer is the most user-friendly on the market—a cinch to figure out and clean.

YOU WANT TO JUICE LIKE A HOLLYWOOD CELEB WITHOUT BUSTING YOUR BUDGET: The Omega J8004, J8005 or J8006 and the Champion Commercial are business-grade machines that juice bars use. Now if you could just get Salma Hayek to come over and show you how to whip up an almond nut milk juice.

YOU HATE CLEANING UP AFTER YOURSELF: You have a life to live, places to go, juices to drink—you don't have time to fiddle with a sink full of different juicer pieces. Hands-down, the Omega 8003, 8004, 8005 and 8006 all rate as easier to clean than any other single-auger unit.

YOU NEED A JUICER AS QUIET AS A BAR ON SUNDAY MORNING: The Hurom HH Elite series is so silent, you'll think it isn't working.

YOU HATE GOING TO THE SUPERMARKET: The Omega VRT400 HDS Juicer with Tap comes with its own organic wheatgrass-growing kit.

YOU WANT A JUICER THAT WORKS HARD FOR THE MONEY: The Samson Matstone 6-in-1 Juicer has six completely different functions at its auger fingertips—you can extract juice from fruit, vegetables and wheatgrass; mince or chop seasonings; mince meats and fish; use it as a food mill to make breadsticks, cookies and pastas; extract oil from sesame seeds (extra attachment required); and whip it out at parties to impress friends and loved ones. Plus it only takes 15 seconds to assemble or disassemble and about a minute to clean!

YOU WANT TO JUICE FOR THE WHOLE FAMILY: The Commercial Champion has a heavy-duty motor that can take lots of abuse and a larger-than-average feeding chute so you can stuff bigger pieces and bigger amounts into the juicer in a shorter amount of time—leaving you more time to ref whose turn it is to control the remote.

YOUR SMART CAR IS BIGGER THAN YOUR KITCHEN: Opt for one of the upright masticators. By flipping the juicing process from horizontal to vertical, you save on countertop and prep space because the feeding chute is also bigger, meaning less need to make big piles of cut-up produce.

YOU LIVE LIFE IN THE FAST LANE: The Kuvings NS-950 Silent Upright Masticating Juicer has a decent pulp catcher so you don't spend half the day straining juice. For real speed, many of the Hurom Slow Juicers are misnomers and almost as fast as centrifugals.

UNLIKE KERMIT, YOU FIND IT EASY BEIN' GREEN: The Solo Star II may not be so sweet on squeezing fruits, but it's super veggie-friendly and does a good job liquefying wheatgrass and leafy vegetables, giving you lots of juice for your green.

Note: This list by no means covers every cold press juicer on the market—use it as a guide to figure out what you're looking for in a cold press juicer.

PIMP YOUR JUICER

Honestly, you don't really need any of these gadgets. That said, you can never be too green or have too many accessories—and they will make prepping, storing and drinking your juice easier.

REALLY GOOD PARING KNIFE: Unlike the chef's knife, which is always used on a cutting board, you can cut with the paring knife while holding it aloft. A quality one will be great for doing everything from peeling fruits and vegetables to slicing a single garlic clove or shallot to removing the ribs from a jalapeño or coring an apple. Most professional cooks use a high-carbon steel, forged knife with a full tang, meaning the blade metal runs from the tip of the knife through the handle to the opposite end.

CUTTING BOARD: Don't settle with just any old wood plank. Look for one that has a handle and a groove (to catch juices) and is dishwasher-safe as well as non-slip.

VEGETABLE BRUSH: You could get a plastic and nylon number from the Dollar Store, but why would you when there are eco- and ergonomic-happy bamboo brushes that fit just so in the palm of your hand, are made with no fertilizers or pesticides, and have fibers that are naturally water-resistant, which inhibits germs and bacteria?

VEGETABLE PEELER: Ideally, you won't be doing much peeling, but if you're worried about pesticides (see "Organic or Conventional?" on page 48) or don't like the look of your carrot, you want to be able to skin it with ease. Look for one with a soft, easy-to-grip handle and swivel blade that lets it move to the contours of whatever you're peeling.

PINEAPPLE CORER: Getting the succulent flesh free of eyes and core could be the hardest thing to love about a pineapple. Different approaches work, but a purpose-made pineapple slicer will do the job in seconds. Good ones resemble mini bicycle pumps; you sink the cutting teeth into a beheaded pineapple and twist the handle to drive the propellerlike cutting blades all the way down to the base. What you pull up, in theory, is a slinky spiral of peeled fruit, picture-perfect for juicing.

CITRUS PEELER: Nothing can make peeling citrus fun, but a dedicated peeler will make it easier.

MEASURING CUPS: You probably have some, but maybe you can't find the half cup or you have dry ingredient cups but none for liquid. It's worth investing in a durable, dishwasher-safe set that includes a two-cup (more useful than you can ever guess) measurement.

REUSABLE PRODUCE BAGS: Those supermarket produce bags are made using oil and are too flimsy to reuse. Invest in a mesh bag—they're lightweight and color-coded so the type A personalities can put their greens in the green bag, their reds in the red bag and so on.

PRODUCE-SAVER DISC: Juicing requires heaps of produce, but if you don't use it all right away, it can rapidly deteriorate. All it takes is one bad apple to spoil the whole bunch—or ethylene (a natural plant hormone released as a gas that triggers cells to degrade), which destroys produce cells. This little gizmo keeps things fresh in your produce drawer for three times longer by absorbing the additional gas.

LETTUCE KEEPER: This actually works on most vegetables and fruit. The water reservoir in the base keeps produce moist for up to two weeks in the fridge and the adjustable venting regulates air circulation and moisture.

MASON JARS: These are great for storing and then grabbing your juice on the go (and looking like you're an official HJ).

INSULATED STAINLESS STEEL BOTTLE/THERMOS: If you tend to be a klutz, this is a sturdier option for juice toting.

COOLER BAG: You'll definitely need a quality thermal bag to keep juice from overheating.

GLASS STRAW: Not necessary, but a plastic-free oh-so-hip way of avoiding a green mustache, these are more durable (and reusable) than paper straws.

SPROUTER: Grow your own sprouts right on your kitchen counter.

FRUIT AND VEGETABLE WASH: Sure, white vinegar and water will also do the trick, but it doesn't feel as official as a soap that's been created simply to remove, as Fit Fruit & Vegetable Wash touts, "...98 percent more pesticides, waxes, people-handling residues and other contaminants versus washing with water alone... leaving no aftertaste or smell: just the taste and nutrition that nature intended."

NUT MILK BAG: Basically, this is a specially shaped fabric bag to strain any remaining pulp or fiber from your almond milk. Of course, you could just use cheesecloth, but then you'd miss out on the fun of telling people you ordered a nut milk bag.

COMPOST CONTAINER: If you're going to keep refuse on your kitchen counter, it should look good. Opt for easy-to-clean stainless steel.

SLAP CHOP: Filed under "Total Indulgence," but this late-night infomercial offering will work like a karate master on your pile of produce, *uchi*-ing it juicing-ready in minutes.

FOOD CO-OP/COMMUNITY SUPPORTED AGRICULTURE (CSA) ASSOCIATION MEMBERSHIP: This one's actually as necessary as it is practical for getting your hands on locally grown, organic or low-pesticide produce in large amounts at affordable prices.

A GARDEN: Of course, you can start your own CSA, too, with your own little corner of green. Lettuce, parsley, broccoli, kale, spinach, basil, carrots and beets (the staples of juice) are a cinch to grow (see "Grow Your Own" on page 52).

CHAPTER THREE
GETTING JUICY

You've made the plunge and bought a cold press juicer. But how do you actually start whipping up those mouthwatering cashew-cacao-apple-mint-kale green concoctions juice bars are so famous for? It turns out that juicing is like most things in life in that there's a right way and most definitely a wrong way to do it. Luckily, while it's easy to make rookie mistakes, it's even easier to follow a few basic steps to start juicing like a Hollywood celeb's chef. Here's everything you need to brew a batch at home and squeeze the most out of your juice.

STEP ONE: GET A RECIPE

If you wing it from Day One and start chucking ingredients into your machine willy-nilly, chances are that the short-term results will be some pretty scummy-looking drinks, a clogged juicer and some choice language; the long-term upshot is that your bright and shiny new appliance may end up gathering dust on the top of your fridge. Recipes are the single best way to elevate your green juice from yuck to yum. They don't just help you create a perfect juice, but they teach you flavor and texture combinations, as well as proper proportions. Once you have a few juices under your belt, you can grab-bag your juicing ingredients. Until then, these guidelines will help you find your perfect mix:

BALANCE IT OUT: The four parts vegetable, one part fruit ratio may be tough to stomach at first as leafy greens can have a bitter taste. Counteract the astringent flavor with a squeeze of lemon, a sprinkle of salt (if not cleansing) or a high-sodium vegetable like celery or carrots, a strong seasoning such as ginger or cinnamon, or a watery produce like apples, cucumber, tomato, celery, grapes, melons and citrus fruit (see "The Five Primary Taste Sensations" on page 45 for more on how to mesh flavors). Those watery fruit and vegetables or an actual splash of liquids like nut milk or water (see "Get Hydrated" on page 60) are also often necessary to add a little fluidity to your juice and stop it from looking and tasting like green sludge.

MAKE IT REAL: It'd seem that the best way to get the most out of juicing is to load up your shopping tote with a whole mess o' greens, greens and more greens, with maybe a few of the antioxidant superfoods thrown in. But you're not going to make juicing a regular habit if you force-feed yourself vegetables you don't smack your lips over in their original whole state. Much better is to ease your taste buds into a greener juice by starting off with ingredients that you already like and then gradually introducing new flavors one by one while eliminating the more sugary ingredients until you've reached the four vegetables to one fruit ratio.

MIX THINGS UP: Juicing over the long run (i.e., your life) is going to be a lot more interesting and also healthier if you shake up your shopping list regularly. Not only will using a variety of ingredients keep your taste buds on their toes, it will ensure that your body is being exposed to the full range of nutrients that veggies and fruits offer.

TASTE WHAT YOU MAKE: To learn how to juice without a recipe safety net, dip your straw in and taste as you press. Even if you're following a tried-and-true method, your apple might be juicier or your grapes more sour or your spices and herbs weaker or your juicer might have less pressing power or Venus might be in retrograde or a million other variables. Your palate is your best control factor.

MATCH FLAVORS: Some vegetables and fruits are the s'mores of the produce world in that they're three distinct flavors that, when combined, are surprisingly delicious. One way to know which ones work well together is to think what you'd want to eat. For instance, melon, garlic and broccoli doesn't sound appetizing, but when you switch out the melon for orange and the garlic for red onion, the dish takes on an entirely different flavor. (Hint: If it sounds like something you'd put together at the salad bar, then it'll probably make an appetizing way to fill your juice glass.)

THE FIVE PRIMARY TASTE SENSATIONS

SALTY: Too much salt may kill us, but our bodies need some of it to survive. The general sodium daily amount to aim for is less than 1,500 mg (about ¾ teaspoon or 3.75 grams) and no more than 2,300 mg (about 1 teaspoon or 6 grams). Surprisingly, salt works better than sugar to suppress bitter tastes, making relatively high-sodium ingredients like chickpeas, celery, Swiss chard, beets, carrots, spinach, artichokes or even a pinch of salt are good green juice choices.

Side note: Salt is the ultimate cooking accessory because it helps showcase the taste of the other ingredients. But if you accidentally over-shake the salt, desalinate with a splash more liquid and a little sweetness.

SWEET: Your yen for sweet things is actually biological. Humans are hardwired to get the quickly digestible calories sugary foods provide. Of course, this was a bit more important back in the days when getting dinner required polishing your spear and tracking woolly mammoths. Luckily, like most things, your sweet tooth mellows with age. Still, a little natural sweetness is what's going to stop your gag reflex from kicking in when you drink up your green juice. Sugar is good at simultaneously promoting other flavors while masking sour and bitter tastes. Fruit is the best source for sugar along with red/orange/yellow peppers and starchy vegetables like parsnips, carrots and beets, but stick to that 4:1 ratio—a little sweetness goes a long way.

Side note: Like salt, sugar brings out the best in all of your other ingredients. But you can have too much sweetness in your juice. To tone it down, add a dash of sour such as a squeeze of lemon or a splash of vinegar.

SOUR: Tart tastes are caused by acids in foods. This is different from bitter, which tends to leave more of a harsh aftertaste (a grapefruit is sour; its rind is bitter). Studies have found that the only mammals with a taste for sour are humans; other animals avoid them. Sour receptors also show up in neurons of the spinal cord, turning the body into a primitive chemical pH tester. In green juices, a little acid helps brighten up flavors and balance out salty, spicy and sweet ingredients. Anything citrus, a dash of vinegar, Granny Smith apples or sour cherries will add some instant oomph.

Side note: If your juice makes you pucker, add some sweetness to cut down on the sour taste.

STRONG/BITTER: Bitter is the only taste that takes some learning to like. Some primitive part of our brain seems to reject bitter tastes by default, probably because many toxic plants taste bitter. Leafy greens like kale, spinach and Romaine lettuce, unsweetened chocolate, broccoli, Brussels sprouts, garlic, onions, dandelion greens and rhubarb are acquired tastes that work better when rounded out with at least one of the four other flavors. If the juice is too sweet or rich-tasting, bitter ingredients such as grapefruit or dark greens can scale it down.

Side note: Salt and sugar will keep bitterness at bay.

SAVORY: This moreish flavor, called umami, is the Johnny-come-lately to the taste world as it was only identified recently. Coined by a Japanese scientist in the early 1900s (the four other tastes had been on the tongue scene for a few thousand years already), it roughly translates as yummy or delicious. Glutamate, an amino acid, has been ID'd as the source of all this moreish wonder. It's naturally present in herbs and spices, tomato, carrots, green tea and cabbage and thought to bring out the essentialness of the other tastes—making your juice more salty/sweet/strong/sour tasting. This is why onions, garlic and mushrooms form an umami *ménage à trois* made in heaven.

Side note: Although umami is rarely a flavor that comes up in juicing, bitter and sours will help when the umami of a drink is overwhelming.

GET GREEN

Three blind mice, the Three Stooges, the three chords used to play every AC/DC song, the three wise men—good things come in threes. The same goes for leafy greens, which have three distinctly different flavors:

1. Lighter-colored lettuce, parsley, spinach, Swiss chard, bok choy, cabbage—mild and goes with anything.

2. Kale, beet and turnip greens, collards—earthy and best with acid and herbs to tone it down.

3. Dandelion greens, cress, mustard, escarole, romaine lettuce, arugula, endive—peppery and you either love it or hate it.

STEP TWO: GET THE BEST INGREDIENTS

Eat fresh, not frozen; eat organic, not conventionally grown; eat raw, not cooked. Eat this: The above isn't necessarily true.

FRESH OR FROZEN?

Don't ice your frozen section just yet—check your calendar first. When vegetables are in season, buy them locally or grow your own (see "Grow Your Own" on page 52 for how to plot your own juicing farm). Off season, head to the freezer section. Freezing is nature's pause button. It helps maintain the nutritional value of fresh vegetables, even during storage. Studies by the Institute of Food Research have shown that produce can lose up to 45 percent of its essential nutrients during the (on average) two weeks it takes to travel from farm to table. During transport, the produce is in a constant state of nutritional deterioration, exposed to pesticides, extreme heat and light. By contrast, most frozen fruits and vegetables are quickly blanched, boiled or steamed and then frozen within hours of being picked, locking in both fresh flavor and nutritional value. Frozen produce is also available year-round and, in most cases, is cheaper than fresh. Choose frozen produce packages marked with a USDA "US Fancy" shield, which signals that the stuff inside is the best in show for size, shape, color and nutrients as opposed to the lower grades "US No. 1" or "US No. 2."

Cold pressing frozen veggies also means you can skip some of the wash, peel and chop prep work, don't have to stress about using your bounty before it spoils and will be able to whip up more flavor combos for less money by opting for mixed vegetable or fruit bags.

These fruits and vegetables have a short shelf or seasonal life and/ or store better in the freezer, so their nutrients and antioxidants stay locked in, making them the best picks for buying iced (Bonus: There's no shell/stalk/pit wastage; you'll use every fiber):

Berries (blueberries, strawberries, raspberries)	Cherries
	Green beans
Broccoli florets	Peaches
Brussels sprouts	Peas, shelled
Butternut squash	Soybeans (edamame), shelled
Carrots	
Cauliflower	Spinach

If using frozen produce, let it thaw a few minutes before juicing. You may need to add more liquid than you usually do as the colder content will give your drink slushy status.

ORGANIC OR CONVENTIONAL?

Your juice is only as clean as what you put in it. You will, for the most part, be drinking your juice ingredients raw, peel and all. So in general, it pays to upgrade and buy organic to avoid getting a mouthful of pesticides. But that doesn't mean you need to splurge for every piece of produce that goes into your green drink. Every year, the Environmental Working Group makes a pesticide analysis of more than 28,000 samples taken by the USDA and FDA to determine which fruits and vegetables have the most bug killers, fungicides and other chemicals. Here's your shopping list based on their most recent ranking, starting from the dirtiest to the cleanest pesticide load:

1. Apples	6. Spinach
2. Strawberries	7. Sweet bell peppers
3. Grapes	8. Nectarines (imported)
4. Celery	9. Cucumbers
5. Peaches	10. Potatoes

11. Cherry tomatoes
12. Hot peppers
13. Blueberries (domestic)
14. Lettuce
15. Snap peas (imported)
16. Kale/Collard greens
17. Cherries
18. Nectarines (domestic)
19. Pears
20. Plums
21. Raspberries
22. Blueberries (imported)
23. Carrots
24. Green beans
25. Tangerines
26. Summer squashes
27. Broccoli
28. Winter squashes
29. Green onions
30. Snap peas (domestic)
31. Oranges
32. Tomatoes
33. Honeydew melons
34. Cauliflower
35. Bananas
36. Watermelons
37. Mushrooms
38. Sweet potatoes
39. Cantaloupes
40. Grapefruits
41. Kiwis
42. Eggplants
43. Asparagus
44. Mangos
45. Papayas
46. Sweet peas (frozen)
47. Cabbages
48. Avocados
49. Pineapples
50. Onions
51. Sweet corn

Note: The produce listed from 37–51 are considered the Clean 15 because they rank at the bottom of the list in terms of pesticide contamination and don't need an organic label to get an uncontaminated bill of health.

RAW OR COOKED?

Some vegetables blanch when confronted with a little heat, while others, especially those containing fat-soluble vitamins like A, D, E and K, need some warming up to release the full blast of their health-boosting nutrients.

Keep It Raw

Eating your food raw means you have a higher risk of food poisoning if you don't prepare your ingredients. See "Get Prepped" on page 66 for fail-safe steps to take before juicing.

ARUGULA: Eating it raw means you'll reap its high B vitamin levels.

BEETS: Cooking can reduce its folate, the B vitamin which may protect against aging of the brain and help prevent cognitive decline by as much as 25 percent.

CRUCIFEROUS FAMILY (BROCCOLI, CABBAGE, BOK CHOY, CAULIFLOWER, WATERCRESS): These veggies contain the enzyme myrosinase, which helps cleanse the liver of carcinogens. Giving them the third degree damages their efficacy.

GARLIC: Heat kills the compound allicin, which is responsible for the antibiotic, antiviral and anti-inflammatory effects of garlic in the body.

GREEN LEAF LETTUCE: Chock-full of the immune-boosting antioxidant, vitamin C, which is easily destroyed by heat.

Heat It Up

Although high temperatures might reduce some of their vitamins and minerals, cooking these vegetables can bring out their antioxidants, raising their overall nutritional value. However, cooking is not another word for boiling to death or frying. A quick, two-minute blanch should provide enough heat to keep vegetables supercharged and fresh-tasting for juicing.

ASPARAGUS: Heat fires up this herbaceous plant's levels of antioxidants, including beta carotene, lutein, lycopene and ferulic acid, which also protect the body against free radicals and may help slow the aging process.

CARROTS: A flash in the water pan increases beta-carotene levels, which, as vitamin A, plays a starring role in vision, reproduction, bone growth and regulating the immune system.

PEPPERS: Cooking can help supply more antioxidants, such as carotenoids and the antioxidant ferulic acid.

TOMATOES: Okay, this is really a fruit, botanically speaking, but the Supreme Court put its two cents in and declared that they can also be considered a vegetable, so case closed. Raw, fresh tomatoes have a total antioxidant potential of about 80; heating them jacks that number up as much as six times, further lowering risk of heart attack and certain cancers upon consumption. Cooking transforms the lycopene into trans-lycopene, which is more readily absorbed by the body.

ZUCCHINI: Zucchini weighs in with five times as much vitamin A, and even a little more folate and niacin, after a hot water dip.

STEP THREE: PICK YOUR PRODUCE

Start with the essentials. The three basic rules for choosing ripe and tasty produce read like a list of bad behavior in a singles bar:

EYE IT: Avoid anything with dark marks, obvious bruises, cracks (especially in root vegetables as they mean it's too dry), dents and/or spots. The freshest flavor is going to come from locally grown produce, even if it's misshapen. Produce in supermarkets needs to travel long distances; they're grown for coming out of a packing case picture-perfect, but aren't always as tasty as they appear.

TIP Head toward the light in the produce display. A study published in the *Journal of Agricultural and Food Chemistry* revealed exposure to continuous light for as little as three days will boost levels of vitamin C and preserve levels of K, E, folate and the carotenoids lutein and zeaxanthin.

GROPE IT: Fruit surfaces will be smooth and even with a firm, but not rock-hard, surface. The flesh should give a little when pressed. Heaviness indicates how juicy fruits like citrus and melon are, but vegetables should be as firm as a three year old's parents.

SNIFF IT: A strong aroma may reveal overripe and past-their-prime fruits. A light, sweet smell is what you want to whiff. Most vegetables don't give you clues to their ripeness by smell the way that fruits do, but you'll know the vaguely stinky smell of slow rot or mold when you sniff it.

GROW YOUR OWN

Of course, you can skip the supermarket altogether and just grown your own. One thing that quickly becomes clear is that you're going to need a lot of produce to sustain your juicing habit. Pounds' worth—which translates to a fat wallet's worth. One way to save some green is to grow some instead.

Most of the vegetables and some of the fruits used for juicing are easy to start sprouting at home, even if your thumb is browner than dirt. That said, many are also easy to find in local nurseries as starter plants. Either way, they should come with specific care instructions. The 18 edibles listed below are a good place to get started on your own homegrown juice garden because they give a lot of bang for their time, energy and knowledge buck. Check "Organic or Conventional?" on page 48 to see if you need to get the official label. If you want to start small, keep buying the cheaper green drink stock items like carrots, beets, apples, celery and cucumbers, and save your sweat and greenbacks to grow the greener stuff that form the nutritional base of juicing—herbs, lettuce, kale, spinach, wheat grass, microgreens, sprouts and other leafy vegetables—at home. Some can even be grown year-round with a little extra care. You'll be reaping your essential juice ingredients before you can say "Mary, Mary, Quite Contrary."

You don't have to get up to your elbows in cow poop to plant your own garden. You can put one in without even picking up a shovel. Just build a raised bed (gardener-speak for a simple frame of rot-resistant lumber, cinder blocks or whatever else you want to use that will make a low wall to hold the soil and your plants), tip some bags of potting soil and compost in, and plant.

TIP Still too much work? Use containers, plastic tubs or even garbage cans to plant. Add drainage holes for the water.

Setting Up Your Garden

DARK, LEAFY GREENS: Collards, kale, cabbage, Romaine lettuce, spinach and Swiss chard are the stars of any green juice. All are cold-weather crops that do best in early spring and fall, but they can last well into winter in snowy regions. If you want a lot, you have to plant a lot. You can harvest by picking the largest leaves when you're ready to eat them or by cutting all the leaves back to leave about one inch of plant in the ground (the plant will grow back several times throughout the season).

ROOT CROPS: Radishes will give your green drink a sharp edge and grow so quickly that they're ready within a month of planting. Parsnips, rutabagas, kohlrabi, carrots and sweet potatoes will all add a sweet tone without ODing on fructose. Don't forget to throw in the edible root greens as well (except for potato, which is in the nightshade family, so its greens are toxic).

MICROGREENS: Leafy greens and herbs that are still babies, microgreens are especially perfect for newbie juicers. Their taste isn't quite as intense as the full-grown versions, but they pack the same nutritional punch. Very pricey to buy, they cost pennies to grow at home. You won't even need a designated garden. They'll grow in any sunny spot in your house. You can use the same broccoli, cabbage, kale, beet, arugula and tatsoi seeds you'd use to plant outside, but designated microgreen seeds come in a handy premixed pack. Sprinkle the seeds over any shallow tray of soil. Even a prepackaged salad box will work if you add drainage holes. The seeds will sprout in a week and can be harvested once the first true leaves unfurl (about another week). Snip right above the soil line. The plants will continue to grow.

SPROUTS: These might just be the easiest veggies to grow. There are the familiar alfalfa, mung and bean sprouts from the far-out sixties—but radish, clover, mustard, garlic, dill, beet, pea, celery, kidney, pinto, navy, soy and sunflower seeds are also a walk in the park to sprout. In general, any plant that has edible stems and leaves can be sprouted (which eliminates tomatoes and most peppers, which are in that toxic nightshade group). However, the conditions that make sprouts so easy to grow are also bacteria nurseries, particularly for E. coli, salmonella and Bacillus cereus. While the only 100 percent guaranteed protection against contamination is to cook the sprouts, it helps to ensure that the seeds you use are from a reputable source and have actually been packaged specifically for home sprouting (as opposed to ground cover or animal feed). You can go high-tech with gadgets made specifically for propagating sprouts, but the simplest, cheapest way takes about five prep minutes, and all you need is a bunch of things you probably already have: a wide-mouthed, quart-sized jar, cheesecloth or even old pantyhose to cover the mouth of the jar, and a rubber band to secure the covering. Start by soaking around three tablespoons of seeds in two inches of water. Store the covered jar in a dark, cool location for 24 hours. Drain (you may need to shake the jar) and put the jar back in its dark place, preferably resting it at an angle so the seeds don't crowd each other, as this can cause a moldy sludge rather than juice-me-now sprouts. The seeds will need to be rinsed several times a day, drained completely each time. The seeds should start sprouting with tiny roots within five days. Rinse and use.

WHEATGRASS: Measure out enough seeds to cover your seed tray. Rinse and then soak overnight in a covered bowl with three times as much water as seeds. Drain and repeat for a total of three overnight soaks. By the last soak, the seeds should have sprouted roots, which will mean they're ready to plant. Drain and spread the seeds in an even layer across a soil-filled, paper towel–lined seed tray that has drainage holes. It's fine if the seeds are touching each other, but make sure there isn't a big pile in one area. Place in a shady area. Keep things as moist as a tropical forest in rainy season. Water lightly and cover with a few moistened sheets of newspaper, and keep spraying the paper and sprouts. It'll take about nine days for the shoots to reach six inches and be ready for harvesting. Cut above the root. Keep watering the wheatgrass to produce a second crop. Harvest that crop once it's mature. Sometimes you'll be three times lucky and get another batch, but it's usually not as tender and sweet as the first two. Empty the seed tray and start the whole process again.

TOMATOES: There are three basic types of tomato plants (tall, bush and dwarf) and within those, thousands of varieties of different colors, sizes and levels of acidity. The easiest to start with are dwarf because they aren't space hogs and can even be plopped into a container and produce a healthy amount of fruit. If you want to play Mama Nature and slow things down when the tomatoes ripen, pick when green and wrap in a paper bag. Adding a banana to the bag will speed things up.

PEPPERS: Pepper choices range from crispy sweet to fiery hot, from big and blocky to long and skinny. These plants are just the ticket for spot planting in empty spaces around the garden or in a container. Green peppers will eventually turn red if left on the plant, but the more pecks of peppers you pick, the more the plant produces.

HERBS: Cilantro, parsley, chives, basil, sorrel, mint and lemon balm are expensive to buy but a cinch to grow and will add continuous flavor to your juice. They can grow in the ground but do just as well in containers (and in the case of mint, better since it has the tendency to conquer whatever growing space it can invade).

ZUCCHINI: All you need is one seed as this plant gives and gives...and gives. The vegetables have lots more actual juice than most and are a great source of vitamin B, potassium and fiber.

ONIONS: Generally, growing onions from sets is easier and more reliable than from seed. The catch is that onions take a long time to mature (about four months) and are fairly inexpensive anyway, so it's your call if they're worth your effort.

PEAS AND BEANS: Both of these vegetables like to grow up, so give them a pole or trellis. The more you pick, the more they produce. Easy peasy.

LETTUCES: Opt for the darker-leaf varieties. You can pull the whole plant or cut leaves as needed. They like shade, so plant in next to taller tomato and bean plants.

BROCCOLI: This vegetable does well in climates with cooler nights and warm days. Since it's frost-hardy, you can plant it twice per season, putting starters in the ground once a couple of weeks before the last frost and again six to eight weeks before the first fall frost.

BRUSSELS SPROUTS: Like slow-motion, hardier versions of broccoli, these sprouts actually taste a bit sweeter when they've been through a touch of frost. Brussels sprouts hate heat and will get bitter and wan in hot, dry weather.

STRAWBERRIES: Store-bought strawberries are a bizarro version of the real thing—they may look like the berry, but they are often tasteless and scentless. A perfectly ripe, homegrown strawberry is unbelievably sweet and fragrant. The perennial plants are surprisingly hardy and can take much abuse. Plant in a sunny spot for years of happy picking.

ASPARAGUS: Plant once, harvest for years: Growing asparagus in a well-maintained bed can provide you with sweet, slender veggies for up to 15 years. Now add up all the money you just saved.

BLUEBERRIES: These berries demand soil quite different from just about every other garden plant. Like an old disciple of Timothy Leary, they thrive on acid—the higher in alkaline the soil, the better the berry. A regular sprinkle of coffee grounds around the base of the bush will give them just the jolt they need.

RASPBERRIES AND BLACKBERRIES: Like strawberries, these fruit are best when homegrown and so hardy they might take over your garden without regular pruning.

THE JUICIEST INGREDIENTS

Try to include a few of these vegetables and fruits when you cold press to pack on the health benefits and make your juice mouthwateringly delicious. Always include something from the dark-green leafy greens and aim for fruit with a low glycemic index (GI). The GI is measurement system ranks foods on a scale from 1 to 100 based on their effect on causing blood sugar to rise—the ideal is to choose those with a GI below 50 so there'll be less impact on your blood sugar levels.

GI of Juicy Fruits and Veggies

Sweet Veggies Choices (aka The 4's in the 4:1 ratio)	GI value
Asparagus	15
Bell peppers	40
Broccoli	15
Celery	15
Cucumbers	15
Dark-green and leafy greens (spinach, collard greens, Swiss chard, kale, mustard greens)	15
Romaine and darker green lettuce	15
Tomatoes	15
The Roots In-Between*	
Beets	50
Carrots	35
Sweet potatoes	70
Sweet Fruit Choices (aka The 1's in the 4:1 ratio)	
Apples	38
Cherries	22
Grapefruits	25
Grapes	46
Oranges (naval)	42
Pears	38
Plums	39
Strawberries	40

* Root vegetables are high in starch, which eventually turns into glucose, making them highly likely to have a big impact on your blood sugar.

Expect one pound of raw produce to yield around one cup or eight ounces of juice, depending on the juicer brand and the water content of the ingredients.

High-starch fruits, such as bananas, papayas, peaches, avocados and fresh figs have soft textures that can clog and may damage some cold pressers. Even if your juicer can handle them, the juice tends to trickle more into what would be defined as nectar as opposed to juice. To be on the safe side, blend these ingredients separately, stirring them into the drink post-press and adding a splash of liquid from the "Get Hydrated" list (page 60) until the juice reaches straw-sucking thickness.

SYNERGIZE YOUR INGREDIENTS

While any 4:1 vegetables to fruit ratio of cold pressed juice will be a healthy choice, some combinations increase the odds of your body absorbing all the disease-fighting, bone-building, health-spiking nutrients you need. Studies show that some fruits, vegetables and even grains are tag-team players and deliver more vitamins and minerals when devoured together than separately. Here are nine powerhouse produce partners that add up to more than the sum of their nutritional parts to make a happier, healthier, smarter, stronger, sexier, more turbo-charged you:

APPLES + ONIONS + BERRIES: Fights allergies, cancer, weight gain, cardiovascular disease, erectile dysfunction, neurological disorders

DARK GREEN VEGETABLES + TOMATOES: Fights blood clots, eye disease, heart disease

GRAINS + BLUEBERRIES: Fights heart disease, cancer

TOMATOES + BROCCOLI: Fights prostate and ovarian cancer

GREEN TEA + LEMON: Fights cancer, cardiovascular disease, high cholesterol

LEAFY GREENS + ALMONDS: Fights heart disease, cataracts, cancer

KALE + LEMON: Fights anemia

LEAFY GREENS + VEGETABLES WITH EDIBLE SKINS: Fights gastrointestinal tract infections and disorders

BERRIES + GRAPES: Fights heart disease

DRINK YOUR COLORS

The fastest way to spot synergy in your juicer—and guarantee a mason jar brimming with doctor-approved goodness—is to make sure your juice recipe has a minimum of three colors. The different pigmentations of fruits and vegetables act as shorthand for the nutritional benefits that they pony up. Yes, it follows that if three colors are good, four are better and so on, but this might be a good time to channel your kindergarten teacher and recall what happens when you have a color-mix free-for-all: You end up with brown. Healthy brown, to be sure, but difficult to gulp down without thinking of other brown-colored things associated with the body. Here's how to crack the nutritional color code:

Orange/Yellow

Code: This produce is brimming with beta-carotene, which muscles up the immune system and eye health.

Juicing Ingredients: Carrots, sweet potatoes, cantaloupe, peaches, apricots, mango, yellow/orange bell peppers, golden/yellow beets, butternut squash.

Green

Code: The diva shade of juicing, anything green means it's loaded with lutein, which keeps eyes healthy by reducing risk of cataracts and macular degeneration, and nutrients like iron, vitamins A, C and K, fiber, protein and antioxidants, which protect against pretty much all cancers and detoxify your body (particularly your liver).

Juicing Ingredients: Leafy greens like kale, collards, lettuce, spinach, cabbage, watercress, Swiss chard, parsley, broccoli, Brussels sprouts, beans, celery, green grapes, kiwis.

Blue/Purple

Code: This dark hue means you have the fountain of youth in one piece of produce—it usually contains anthocyanins, flavonoids and antioxidants that boost brain health, improve circulation, protect against arthritis and act as anti-aging agents.

Juicing Ingredients: Blackberries, blueberries, red grapes, plums, red cabbage.

White/Tan

Code: Usually associated with evil, processed foods like white bread and table sugar, these whites are the superheroes of the produce world, fighting against viral, fungal and bacterial infections.

Juicing Ingredients: Onions, garlic, apples, squashes, cauliflower.

Red

Code: Sometimes called the new green for all the health goodies these tinted foods offer up, including reducing the risk of several types of cancer, particularly prostate; improving workouts by helping your body use oxygen more efficiently and aiding in muscle recovery; lowering blood pressure; and acting as an aphrodisiac by boosting testosterone and bolstering brain power.

Juicing Ingredients: Tomatoes, watermelons, pink grapefruits, red bell peppers, cherries, raspberries, red apples.

SECRET INGREDIENTS TO JUICE THINGS UP

These superfood smart bombs will power up your juice—but a little goes a long way. A tablespoon per eight ounces of juice should be enough to boost your drink. *Note:* If your juicer doesn't have a separate function for seeds like chia, flax and sesame, grind them in a blender first or just stir in whole to finished juice.

SMOOTH-WORKING FIBER: Chia seeds, maca powder, flaxseed

POTENT JOLT OF PROTEIN: Spirulina powder, chlorella powder, nuts and/or seeds (sunflower, pumpkin, sesame, chia, flax, hemp powder), carob powder, lucuma powder, bee pollen

GUT SCRUBBER: Miso paste, chlorella, probiotic powder, garlic, mint, kombucha (see "Skip Store-Bought and Get Self-Sufficient" on page 61 for how to make your own mother lode)

RDA OF VITAMINS AND MINERALS: Maca powder (B12, iron, calcium), lucuma powder (potassium, magnesium, phosphorus), cacao powder (antioxidant, magnesium), carob powder (potassium, calcium), nutritional yeast flakes (vitamins B12, B1, B2, B3, B6, folic acid, pantothenic acid, zinc and selenium)

HEALTHY FAT: Coconut (meat, oil, butter), nuts and/or seeds (sunflower, pumpkin, sesame, chia, flax, hemp powder), maca powder

LOW-GI/GL SWEET TOOTH SATISFACTION: Honey, stevia leaf powder or extract, Medjool date syrup (see the following page for recipe), lucuma powder, liquid herbals or tinctures, bee pollen, cacao powder, vanilla bean powder, agave, yacon syrup, brown rice syrup, barley malt syrup.

Note: Although these sweet alternatives have a low GI/GL, many still pile on calories, so use sparingly.

BLOOD SUGAR STABILIZING/DE-CLOTTING SPICES: Cinnamon, turmeric, fenugreek seeds, chile peppers

GUT SOOTHERS: Ginger, cinnamon, peppermint, chamomile

IMMUNE-SYSTEM PROTECTING HERBS AND SPICES: garlic, turmeric, ginger, thyme, chili pepper

GET HYDRATED

If you only have a few pounds of produce, have produce with low water content, or are simply in the mood for a thinner juice, add a splash of liquid. Of course, water will do, but these nourishing potions add flavor along with flow to your cup of goodness.

COCONUT WATER: This is the liquid inside young green coconuts, not the milk that comes from cold pressing the meat. A study in *Medicine & Science in Sports & Exercise* gave this sweet, nutty, potassium-loaded liquid a seal of approval for replenishing body fluids just as well as sports drinks—and even better than water.

NUT MILK: Although it has a low GI, it's a sweet way to add some liquid protein to your juice.

SPROUTED GRAIN MILK: Although non-dairy, it'll give your juice a creamy shot of live enzymes, low GI carbs, fiber and protein. If you use oats, you'll be doubling down with a blast of sweet flavor.

ALOE VERA JUICE: Because of its gelatinous texture and instability, it's better to buy than make cactus juice. Know that the research isn't conclusive on health benefits—on one side, it may help in some digestive conditions and on the other, aloe vera juice (specifically the kind containing aloin), may be linked to higher cancer risk.

SOY MILK: High vitamin D, calcium and protein levels mean this is the only non-dairy milk that can go nose-to-nose with cow milk, so a splash will transform your juice into a (soy) milk shake.

RICE MILK: High in sweetness and low in just about everything else, including gluten, lactose and protein, a rice milk base will take the bitter edge off of a green juice.

KOMBUCHA TEA: Unlike your grannie's Earl Grey, this tea will add a fizzy dose of probiotics to your juice, turning it into a salubrious soda substitute.

SKIP STORE-BOUGHT AND GET SELF-SUFFICIENT

Make your own hydrating liquids from scratch. Here are some quick-and-easy recipes, from the department of saving money:

MEDJOOL DATE SYRUP

Makes about 1 cup of syrup

10 whole Medjool dates

3 cups water

2 teaspoons lemon juice (acts as natural preservative)

dash of ground cinnamon (optional)

Soak the dates in 1½ cups of water for an hour. Drain and pit. Blend the pitted, rehydrated dates with the remaining 1½ cups of water, lemon juice, and cinnamon on high for 1 minute until smooth. Refrigerate for up to 3 weeks in an airtight container.

NUT/SEED MILK

Makes about 2 cups

> 1 cup raw nuts/seeds
>
> 6 cups water

Soak nuts/seeds in 2 cups of water overnight (or for 8 hours). Adjust your cold press juicer so the juicing screen and position bowls are under the bottom and end spouts. Drain the nuts/seeds and add the remaining 4 cups of water. Scoop the nuts and water mix into the pressing section. The liquid will be strained and the fibrous material will exit out of the end spout. Continue until all nuts/seeds have been ground and pressed. Re-press the ground nut/seed pulp to extract all of the juice. Save nut/seed pulp in an airtight container in the fridge (use within 3 days) or freezer for cooking or add it to your juice for more protein.

SPROUTED GRAIN MILK

Makes about 4 cups

> 1 cup grain (wheat, kamut, quinoa, amaranth, millet, teff, spelt or rolled oats)
>
> 6 cups water

Soak the grains in 2 cups of water for 8 hours or overnight. Rinse and, to sprout, leave at cool room temperature for 24 hours. Blend with 4 cups of water until smooth. Strain through fine nut milk bag (may need to do this twice to completely drain) and store in an airtight container for up to 5 days. Stir before using. Keep the pulpy mush for baking or eating or mixing back into your juice for a thicker drink.

SOY MILK

Makes about 5 quarts of milk

    1 cup dried soy beans

    12 cups water

Soak the beans in 4 cups of water for 8 hours or overnight. Drain, rinse and press in your juicer. Add 8 cups of water to the mashed beans and press through the juicer again. Strain the liquid through a fine nut milk bag. There's controversy over whether raw soybeans cause gastric problems including diarrhea, vomiting and possibly death. To be on the safe side, low-simmer the resulting pressed milk for around 25 minutes, stirring regularly. Store for up to 5 days in an airtight container in the fridge.

BROWN RICE MILK

Makes about 4 cups

    1 cup brown rice

    8 cups water

Cook the rice in the water until it's really soft. Let cool, or refrigerate, and then cold press it. Stir the pulp into your juice for a thicker drink, eat as a porridge or use to bake with (store the pulp in an airtight container in the fridge for up to 3 days).

COCONUT "MILK" WATER

Makes about 1 cup

> 1½ cups water
>
> 1 cup dry, unsweetened shredded or flaked coconut (you can use a fresh coconut, but it's time-consuming and finger-risking to de-flesh)

Juice the coconut, then cover the pulp with water, letting it sit for 8 hours or overnight. Re-juice it to get a creamy milk. Stir the pulp back into the drink to make it even creamier or store in an airtight container in the fridge (for up to 5 days) or freeze (for up to 2 months) to use for cooking or baking.

KOMBUCHA TEA

Makes about 1 gallon

Use a sweetener such as organic sugar or evaporated cane juice because the "tea" breaks down the sugar and transforms it into acids, vitamins, minerals, enzymes and carbon dioxide—which gives kombucha its signature fizz—and works best with sugar that is more refined and has a mild flavor.

> 2 quarts water
>
> ½ cup sweetener
>
> 4 bags black tea or 1 tablespoon loose black tea
>
> 1 cup unpasteurized, neutral-flavored starter kombucha (available from natural foods stores)
>
> 1 SCOBY (Symbiotic Colony of Bacteria and Yeast), aka "mother" or "mushroom" (available from natural food stores or begged from a kombucha pal)

Boil the water with the sweetener until it's dissolved. Add the tea. Steep until the water has cooled (a bowl of ice under the pot will speed things up). Strain out the tea. Stir in the starter kombucha. Transfer to a large glass jar and add the SCOBY. Cover the mouth of the jar with a few layers of cheesecloth or paper towels secured with a rubber band. Leave in a dark area at room temperature for a week, checking occasionally.

The SCOBY may float to the top or sink to the bottom. A new, cream-colored layer of SCOBY should start forming on the surface within a few days. It might attach to the old SCOBY or separate. There may also be unappetizing-looking, brown stringy bits floating beneath the SCOBY, sediment collecting at the bottom, and/or bubbles collecting around the SCOBY, which are gross but actually all signs of healthy fermentation.

After seven days, start taste testing the kombucha daily. When it's your perfect blend of tart and sweet, it's ready to bottle. First prepare and cool another pot of strong tea for your next batch of kombucha, as outlined above. Then lift out the SCOBY and put it on a clean plate. Measure out 1 cup of starter tea from the previous batch and add to the just-brewed tea. Put this aside for now.

Strain the fermented kombucha into bottles, leaving about ½ inch of head room in each bottle, and store at room temperature in a dark cool place for up to 3 days for kombucha to carbonate. Refrigerate to stop fermentation and carbonation and use within 1 month.

To brew the next batch, combine the starter tea from your last batch of kombucha with a fresh amount of sugary tea and pour it into the cleaned fermentation jar. Slide the SCOBY on top, cover and ferment for the 7 to 10 days. Even if you're not brewing up more tea, you'll still need to feed and care for your SCOBY (it's like a goldfish). It can last a long time if stored in a fresh batch of the tea base with the starter tea in the fridge. Change out the tea for a fresh batch every 4 to 6 weeks and peel off the bottom (oldest) layer every few batches (this is your stash for passing on to kombucha-brewing wannabes).

STEP FOUR: GET PREPPED

Don't even be tempted to skip this section—most juicing ingredients are consumed raw, which, according to the FDA, means that they're more at risk of harboring pathogens responsible for cyclosporiasis, E. coli, hepatitis, salmonellosis and bacillary dysentery. All produce, including organic, is grown in dirt and manhandled by many people before it ends up in your juicer. Properly cleaning and storing it means you still reap all the vitamins, minerals, fiber and disease-protecting benefits without the risk.

But here's some good news for procrastinators—prepping your produce for juicing is all about putting it off until tomorrow. You need to wait until the produce is ripe before using it, you need to wait until you're going to use it to wash it (storing may promote bacterial growth and speed up spoilage) and you need to wait until you've washed it to prepare it for juicing. The only thing you need to do right away is put it away.

STORING YOUR PRODUCE

The question of storage seems to divide produce into three camps: Produce that thrives in room temperature, produce that prefers cellarlike conditions and produce that does best in cool, moist air. You don't have to memorize the list below; just picture how the produce is displayed at the supermarket for a quick mental guide.

TIP Produce likes to be segregated. Keep everything in separate bags to avoid high-ethylene fruits rubbing up and spoiling other items and strong-smelling vegetables contaminating all the other produce.

PRODUCE THAT THRIVES IN ROOM TEMPERATURE: This type of produce is easy—just leave them on the counter. The likes of non-cherry stone fruits, tomatoes, mangos, melons, apples, kiwis and pears will continue to ripen when left at room temperature. In fact, the USDA has found that watermelon, tomatoes and peaches continue to develop nutrients (including the phytochemicals lycopene and beta-carotene) after picking if they're kept at room temperature rather than chilled in a fridge.

TIP To speed ripening, paper-bag the fruit/vegetable to concentrate the release of ethylene. To turbo-charge the process, throw in a high-ethylene-producing food, such as a banana or an apple.

Note: Soft fruits like peaches and bananas can clog juicers and, depending on your juicer, should be used sparingly if at all. The juice from these fruits is very thick and closer to nectar than thin juice.

PRODUCE THAT PREFERS CELLARLIKE CONDITIONS: Winter squashes, potatoes, onions and garlic fall into this group.

PRODUCE THAT DOES BEST IN COOL, MOIST AIR: Put bell peppers, zucchini, grapes, green onions, peas, broccoli, Brussels sprouts, cauliflower, beans, leafy greens and lettuce in individual plastic or produce bags wrapped loosely in a damp paper towel to keep them perky. Cut ¼ inch from the bottom stalks of fresh celery and asparagus and store upright in a little water. Fresh herbs stay crisp behind the leaves when stored in a glass of water lightly covered with a plastic bag. Bag citrus in plastic. Pick over your berries and cherries, chucking any that show the slightest sign of spoilage as the mold will quickly spread to other berries. Store them in as few layers as possible (putting them on paper towels will absorb any excess moisture). Remove tops from root veggies like beets, turnips, radishes and carrots (to keep them from sapping nutrients from the roots; some vegetables will even grow new greens after their tops have been removed) and store separately in plastic bags with a damp paper towel to keep them from wilting. Keep the roots in a water bath or plastic bags wrapped loosely with a damp paper towel. Put sprouts in a bowl of lemon water covered with plastic.

TIP Wilted greens can often be revived by placing them in a dish filled with cold water and refrigerating overnight.

EAT CLEAN WITH CLEAN VEGGIES

Most produce—including melons, cucumbers, winter squashes, citrus and sweet potatoes—can be effectively cleaned under running water. Afterward, give your produce a quick brush with a veggie scrubber (if this seems one step too many, take a moment to imagine how many hands touch the produce before it gets to your mouth). For an extra layer of safety, remove the outer leaves of heads of lettuce and cabbage. If your greens are bagged and marked "ready-to-eat," the FDA may say it's safe to eat without rewashing, but widespread instances of food-poisoning linked to these so-called ready-to-eat foods seems enough of an argument to give them a spritz.

KNIFE SKILLS 101

The one downside of cold pressing your produce is that the auger mechanism requires more knife skills than a centrifugal slice and dice would. However, what you lose in time, you more than make up for in maintaining nutritional content. Here's what you need to get the following produce faves ready to go down the chute:

BUNCH OR ROLL

- ○ Leafy greens

- ○ Sprouts

- ○ Wheatgrass

- ○ Herbs

CHOP INTO PIECES (small enough to easily fit through feeding tube)

- ○ Broccoli

- ○ Bok choy

- ○ Cabbage

- ○ Cauliflower

- ○ Celery

- ○ Cucumbers

- ○ Fennel

- ○ Ginger

- ○ Peppers (deseeding not necessary unless it's a hot pepper)

- ○ Root vegetables such as carrots, radishes, beets, turnips and parsnips (remove greens to add separately)

○ Strawberries (stemming not necessary)

○ Sweet potatoes

○ Tomatoes

CHOP AND CORE/SEED/STONE

○ Apples

○ Cherries

○ Mangos (the peel may jam up the gears)

○ Melons

○ Peaches

○ Pears

○ Plums

PEEL AND CHOP

○ Citrus (leaving as much as the white part as you can)

○ Kiwis

○ Pineapples

○ Pomegranates

○ Squashes

SOAK AND RINSE

○ All nuts should be soaked in water for about 12–24 hours, then rinsed thoroughly before juicing. Feed them into the juicer simultaneously with water.

GRIND

○ Seeds, grains or legumes usually need grinding before adding to a cold press juicer

WHAT COUNTS?

The nine-a-day equation is not as simple as it sounds. In this case, a rose will not smell as sweet by any other name and a carrot is not going to measure up to a cucumber as a single serving. For sticklers who need to know everything down to the last "g" of a milligram, see "Measuring Up" on page 71 for what a single serving is for most fruits and vegetables that might end up in your juicer. For everyone else, here's a cheat sheet rounding up popular produce portion sizes:

Produce Portion Sizes

Ingredient	Such As . . .	Single Serving
Very large fruits	Melons, watermelons, pineapples	1 large slice
Large fruits	Grapefruits, mangos	1 half a fruit
Medium fruits	Apples, oranges, peaches, pears	1 whole fruit
Small fruits	Apricots, clementines, kiwis, passion fruits, plums	2 whole fruits
Berry-type fruits	Blackberries, black currants, blueberries, cherries, cranberries, grapes, raspberries, strawberries	1 mug-size cupful
Mixed salad vegetables	Celery, cucumbers, iceberg and other pale lettuces	1 dessert bowlful
Cruciferous vegetables	Broccoli, Brussels sprouts, cabbage, cauliflower, radishes, turnips	1 small plateful
Green leafy vegetables	Chard, dark-green winter cabbage, kale, bok choy, Romaine lettuce, spinach, watercress	1 small plateful
Medium vegetables	Peppers, tomatoes	1 whole vegetable
Other vegetables	Carrots, green beans, onions, peas, squashes	1 small plateful
Grasses and sprouting beans	Wheatgrass, alfalfa, bean sprouts, millet, mung, rice, oat	½ mug-size cupful

Here's the USDA breakdown of 1 portion (or ½ cup) of fruit and vegetables:

Fruits

- ○ Apple: ½ of a large or 1 small
- ○ Apricot: 1 small
- ○ Cherries: 8 large
- ○ Grapefruit: 1 medium
- ○ Grapes: 16
- ○ Kiwi: 1 small
- ○ Mango: 1 medium
- ○ Melon: 1 slice or ¼ of a medium melon
- ○ Orange: ½ of a large or 1 small
- ○ Pear: ½ of a large or 1 small
- ○ Pepper: 1 large
- ○ Plum: 1 small
- ○ Raspberries: 8 large
- ○ Satsuma/clementine: 1 small
- ○ Strawberries: 8 large
- ○ Tomato: 1 medium
- ○ Watermelon: 1-inch-thick wedge or 6 melon balls of watermelon

Vegetables

- ○ Broccoli: 5 large spears
- ○ Cabbage: 1 cup shredded
- ○ Celery: 2 large stalks
- ○ Carrots: 10 baby or 2 medium
- ○ Lettuce or raw leafy greens such as spinach, Romaine lettuce, watercress, endive or escarole: 1 cup

STEP FIVE: DRINK UP

One of the kickbacks of drinking at home is that you can get a cold-off-the-presses juice buzz within minutes of making your drink without having to fork over part of your paycheck for the pleasure. So swallow your juice as soon as possible. This doesn't mean that you should act like a contestant in a drink-chugging contest. Take your time savoring each mouthful, but remember that it's best to drink your cold press juice within 20 minutes (See "The Best Time to Drink Your Cold Press Juice" on page 80) and, at worst, not to let it sit around for more than a few hours. The older drink may be less vitamin-dense due to oxidation, but it'll still have more nutritional value than just about any other drink—save a fresh-press juice.

Another option for stocking up on juice is to freeze it ASAP after making. Store it in freezer-proof single-serve containers so you can just grab and run. But even frozen isn't forever—try and drink your stash within two weeks of freezing.

If you're taking your juice out for a day trip, make sure you store it in a cooler or take it straight from the freezer to naturally defrost throughout the day.

It isn't more or less healthy to drink your juice along with other foods or after a meal, but your drink will be more quickly digested if it's the only thing in the stomach.

TIP Don't chuck the pulp! Run it through a few times to squeeze every last drop and then flip over to page 186 for what to do with the leftover mush.

JUICER TROUBLESHOOTING

GET UNCLOGGED

Juicing is intended to make you healthier, but one way it can give you a headache is when the juicer clogs. "When" rather than "if" because it will clog. It doesn't matter how expensive the machine is or how many self-cleaning accessories it comes with. And when it clogs, the whole operation grinds to a halt. While you probably won't be able to prevent your juicer from clogging altogether, there are some precautions you can take to make it a rare rather than a regular occurrence:

KEEP IT CLEAN: Yes, you just spent the last 45 minutes of your life making your juice and now all you want to do is drink it and get on with experiencing your health rush. But if you don't at least rinse off the parts, all that leftover vegetable and fruit gunk will harden and require a few more calcium-rich kale and omega-3–rich cauliflower juices to build up the muscle power to scrape your juicer squeaky clean. Make sure you unplug the machine before breaking out the sponge.

If your juicer comes with a pulp bin, line it with biodegradable bag or waste bag. This one-minute extra step will save you the five minutes of cleaning and cussing time it takes to clean this part and makes it easier to collect the pulp for other uses (see page 186 for how to deal with the pulp).

Take the ten extra minutes to wash the juicer parts and throw them in the dishwasher. Even so-called self-cleaning juicers need more than a rinse to keep things cranking along smoothly. While it's okay to let it soak until you can get to it, try not to let vegetable and fruit residue harden on the parts, and make sure you remove all of the pulp in the pulp container.

AVOID TROUBLE: The size of the produce and the order in which you put the cut pieces through the feeder chute can also stop up the works. Keep everything uniformly small—think the size of a grape. Soft fruits and vegetables and anything leafy tend to be the troublemakers. If you regularly run into a jam, start mincing your leafy veggies—about ⅛-inch pieces should be enough to break things up. Alternate between hard and soft; throw in parsnip and carrot pieces, then soft fruit or leafy greens and then hard again. This will help to continually clean out the residue of less firm stuff. Finish the session by running a hard vegetable through the juicer to clean it out (this will make the washing step less messy as most of the residue ends up in your juice or the pulp as opposed to being left in the auger).

OPT FOR FRESHNESS: The older the produce, the more flabby and soft it tends to be—and the more likely it'll gum up the works in your juicer.

GET CENTERED: It's tempting to push things along, especially with cold press machines. But there's a reason they are aka slow pressers. The whole point is that they keep the integrity of the ingredients by rotating slowly and minimizing heating. So take a deep breath, find your inner Zen and let your masticator do what it does best.

WATCH YOUR FIBROUS INGREDIENTS: Some fruit, like pineapple, and some vegetables, such as celery, are more than usual suspects when it comes to backing up your juicer. What they have in common are tough, long fibers.

Produce that falls in this category—asparagus is another culprit—should be chopped small before feeding into the juicer chute and alternated with non-fibrous plants.

STAY VIGILANT: Regularly checking the pulp outlet chute to make sure that the waste pulp is being ejected will give you a heads-up if there's blockage somewhere. If the output slows or is uneven, stop and investigate.

EASY FIXES TO COMMON JUICING SLIP-UPS

Slip-ups while juicing are to be expected, especially if you're new to the game. Luckily, most are a cinch to fix with a few simple tweaks to your technique.

SLIP-UP: You skewed the 80:20 percent vegetable to fruit ratio to something more like 50 percent fruit. Green juices definitely consist of the kind of taste that grows on you. The temptation, at first gag, is to load up on the sweeter flavors to mask some of the greener ones. But fructose is not your friend. The ultimate bad effects from having too much sugar counterbalance anything good you are trying to do for your health by juicing in the first place.

Get It Right: If you do find it hard to swallow the 80:20 percent ratio, add a lemon or lime to your daily concoction, as they're low in sugar and high on flavor. See "The Five Primary Taste Sensations" on page 45 for an at-a-glance guide to balancing the flavors in your drink.

SLIP-UP: Your green juice is too green. Yes, there is such a thing as too much green. Green leafy vegetables like kale, spinach, broccoli, collards and watercress have high goitrogen content. These naturally occurring substances can slow down thyroid function, putting you at greater risk for hypothyroidism.

Get It Right: To keep your juice green and your thyroid healthy, balance out the goitrogen veggies with risk-free exceptions like Romaine, parsley, dandelion greens, cucumber, celery and fennel.

SLIP-UP: You sub out your meals for green juices. A green drink can only be a complete meal if you're adding protein and fiber. Otherwise, it's a supersimple, effective way to get your daily nine for the day but not your RDA of everything else.

Get It Right: To make it meal-worthy, throw in some supplements (see "Secret Ingredients to Juice Things Up" on page 59 for ideas to muscle up your drink).

SLIP-UP: You pressed yucca, rhubarb, raw legumes and/or the pits/seeds of apples, mangos, peaches, pears or apricots. Yucca or cassava root contains cyanide—to make it edible, it first needs to be dried, soaked in water, rinsed and cooked. Rhubarb leaves contain insanely high levels of a toxin called oxalic acid which, when consumed, can cause serious kidney damage, and possibly even death. Even a small amount can make you sick, and 10 or so pounds is enough to kill you. Dried beans contain compounds that inhibit healthy enzyme function and, occasionally, house toxins that cause an upset stomach. Cooking, soaking in water or sprouting the beans destroys these compounds. Stone fruit seeds and pits contain a cyanide compound of which just a tiny amount can cause some serious, if not actually fatal, health risks. Apple and pear seeds contain cyanide in smaller amounts, but still aren't a good idea to regularly juice (citrus seeds also have cyanide, but in less toxic amounts).

Get It Right: Just pour your drink down the drain and start again.

SLIP-UP: Being boring. It's easy to get so wrapped up in the green ingredients that you forget that there's a Skittles rainbow of colors you can add to your drink.

Get It Right: See "Drink Your Colors" on page 58 for a color chart of what makes a (mostly) balanced green drink.

SLIP-UP: Sticking with the kale-spinach one-two punch.

Get It Right: These are good places to start, but your palate will start yawning pretty rapidly if all you give it to drink is kale, kale and more kale, with some spinach thrown in as a flavor burst. There's a world o' leafy greens out there including parsley, cilantro, Swiss chard, dandelion greens, lettuce, collard greens, carrot tops, beet tops, cabbage, mustard greens, tatsoi and bok choy.

SLIP-UP: You added an avocado/banana/papaya/peach/avocado/fresh fig to your drink.

Get it Right: These dense choices can clog your machine and mostly go straight to the pulp. If you really want to have these ingredients in your juices, blend or food process them first and then add other pressed juice to them.

CHAPTER FOUR
CLEAN UP YOUR ACT

Juicing, cleansing and juice cleansing may seem the same, but they are more like one of those transformer bots than interchangeable thesaurus terms. You can juice and you can cleanse and you can go on a (preferably cold press) juice cleanse. Juicing simply means that you drink juice as a supplement to your regular diet or perhaps in place of a meal occasionally. Cleansing is when you eliminate most or all food from your daily diet (you might still have some solids but cherry pick out Diet Destroyers—aka DDs—like alcohol, nicotine, fats, dairy, caffeine, processed and/or refined foods, sugars, gluten and/or animal protein). Stricter cleanses lean more toward liquidating your daily menu, replacing all meals and snacks with a fluid. In a juice cleanse, that fluid will be around 64 ounces of fresh cold press juices for as little as one or as long as seven days. Longer is not recommended, as your body wants, expects, deserves and needs the amount of protein and fiber you really can only get from food to run optimally—drinking juice and nothing but juice for more than a week can end up being counterproductive as your body, in search of energy, slows down its metabolism rate and starts to feed off muscle mass. The longer-term dangers are difficult-to-reverse muscle and bone loss, electrolyte imbalances, malnutrition, organ damage, risk of high cholesterol and digestive problems, to name just a few. So when it comes to juice cleansing, you really can have too much of a good thing.

While there's no hard scientific evidence that a cold press juice cleanse, or any cleanse, for that matter, will flush toxins from your body's personal detoxifying system (your liver, kidney and colon), you do need a balanced diet consisting of minimally processed, nutrient-dense foods to keep those organs functioning at peak performance. So although doctors, scientists and nutritionists are still duking it out over whether there's anything to health claims that any type of cleanse will give you Spock-like mental clarity, force-field your immune system and add a zip to your step and a twinkle to your eye, most agree that chugging heavy-on-the-vegetables juice for one day, three days or even a week will certainly make you feel more energetic and less bloated in the short-term because you're staying away from the DD ingredients that have been shown to cause water retention and late afternoon sluggishness and encourage overeating.

In this context, a juice cleanse is really a way of detoxing your daily diet rather than your body. You reboot your palate and shift yourself away from bad eating habits by eliminating the foods you don't need or want and giving your body easily digestible, tasty, healthy nutrition in their place.

But before you chuck all the food from your pantry and jump on the cleansing bandwagon (along with the aforementioned Salma Hayek, who has started her own green juice line, Owen Wilson, Blake Lively, Alicia Silverstone, Megan Fox, Gwyneth Paltrow, Miranda Kerr, Nicole Richie, Russell Simmons, Ryan Seacrest and Bill Clinton, to name just a few A-listers, are regularly photographed with a big gulp of green juice in tow), but remember that although a cold press juice cleanse is an effective psychological jump-start to healthy eating, being healthy is not a single one-, three- or seven-day event. It's a lifestyle. So the long-term solution is to cold press juice cleanse occasionally and drink cold press juices regularly by supplementing rather than substituting solid foods (including whole fruits and vegetables) in your daily diet. In other words, juice snack. The Harvard-based Nurses' Health Study found that adults who had the highest intake of produce in both solid and liquid form—about eight servings per day—were 30 percent less likely to have a heart attack or stroke than those who got 1.5 or fewer servings daily. Plus, their overall risk for any type of chronic disease was 12 percent lower than that of the fruit and veggie skimpers.

Bear in mind that successfully cleansing your lifestyle is like so many things in life (meeting your soul mate, launching a start-up, throwing the winning pass, achieving simultaneous orgasms, playing the stock market, to name a few): Timing is everything.

TIMING IS EVERYTHING: PROPERLY PLAN A SUCCESSFUL CLEANSE

Proper planning can make all the difference between a successful cleanse and one that ends in failure. Before you chop a single carrot, find out the best time to do everything while cleansing.

THE BEST TIME TO STOP EATING

The impulse can be, "OMG, I just spent the last 72 hours pigging out; I need to go on a cleanse now!" Bad idea. Purposefully bingeing on a few or more of your favorite foods the day before cleansing is also a no-no. Your cleanse starts before you actually start your cleanse. In other words, you need to ease into a cleanse by preparing your body. To help scale down withdrawal symptoms, start your prep work, at minimum, the number of days you intend to cleanse before the actual red letter day. So if you're planning a 24-hour blitz, cut the junk at least a day before, clean up your act three days prior to a 72-hour cleanse cycle and give yourself seven days to prepare for a one-week cleanse.

Prime yourself; the more you can do of the following before starting your cleanse, the more likely you are to have a no-sweat, no-hassle, no-fail experience:

○ Simplify your menu plan (see "Clean Eating" on the following page for what to cross off your shopping list).

○ Substituting one fresh cold press juice for one meal or snack for a few days will help prepare your body for what's in store.

○ Eat the foods you'll be drinking during your cleanse.

○ Up your water intake (see "The Best Time to Drink Other Liquids" on page 81).

○ Cut down on portion sizes so you won't go into hunger overdrive.

CLEAN EATING

Quit these foods* at least five days before and five days after a cold press juice cleanse:

ALCOHOL: switch to nonalcoholic, unsweetened beverages, accompanied by a stress-releasing exercise such as yoga

COFFEE: switch to decaffeinated green or herbal tea

ALL-WHITE SUGAR AND PRODUCTS CONTAINING IT: cookies, cakes, candy, cereals, packaged foods; switch to unprocessed sugar, such as honey or stevia

PROCESSED FOODS: this includes packaged foods, crackers, chips, salty snacks, etc.; switch to fruit and vegetables

WHITE FLOUR: switch to whole wheat

FRIED FOODS: switch to roasting instead

PROCESSED MEATS: salami, hot dogs, lunch meats, sausage; switch to unprocessed versions of the same meat

*Try to eliminate or at least minimize these "foods" and cooking methods from your life altogether.

BEWARE DOWN THERE

Doing anything that messes with your colon (enema, irrigation, hydrotherapy, over-the-counter laxatives) will not jump-start your cold press juice cleanse and may give you a one-way ticket to the emergency room. Studies have linked these procedures with parasitic infections, development of abscesses in the digestive tract, perforation of the rectum and colon, and heart failure due to electrolyte imbalances (brought on by the absorption of excessive amounts of fluid during the colon cleansing procedure). Plus, these kinds of purges can actually disturb healthful bacterial (probiotic) populations in the gut, which are needed for proper digestion and immunity.

THE BEST TIME TO START YOUR (JUICER) ENGINES

Not when you're in the middle of planning a wedding or have a work project due or are in any other way time-crunched. Chopping and cold pressing all that produce takes time, especially if you're a juicing newbie, so block off days in your calendar when you don't need to get up and rush out the door like a sprinter training for the New York City Marathon.

Weekends are an especially good time to start getting your juicing chops, as you'll be able to take five to figure out what happens when you push this button or that lever on your new appliance, concoct new recipes or simply refresh with a midday nap. Plus you may need to spend more time than usual on the throne.

THE BEST TIME TO DRINK YOUR COLD PRESS JUICE, PART ONE

ASAP. As time-efficient as it might seem to whip up a large batch of juice and keep it for a few days, it isn't nutrient effective. The picosecond you juice, every cell wall of the produce is like a nudist at a beach party and completely exposed to air. This causes oxidation (a fancy way of saying that the air is causing their enzymatic and nutritional values to deteriorate). To fortify all the good stuff in your cold press juice, try to drink it within 20 minutes. Lickety-split drinking is also safer, according to the Mayo Clinic, as there is an increased vulnerability to bacteria when fresh unpasteurized juice is stored.

If you really must bolt before you're done, then transfer the liquid to a dark airtight container in the fridge and add a few teaspoons of lemon juice to prevent discoloration. To minimize deterioration, fill it to the brim so there is no extra air space (add water until it levels off before the top).

THE BEST TIME TO DRINK YOUR COLD PRESS JUICE, PART TWO

ASAP. In this case, ASAP stands for "As Slow As Possible." You should take about as long to drink the juice as you did to make the drink in the first place. There are a couple of reasons for this (aside from simply looking like you haven't been raised by wolves). It takes roughly 20 minutes for the brain to send out a "Stop Eating! You're Full!" APB. Add this to the fact that studies show the body's mechanisms for controlling hunger and thirst are completely different, so fluid calories don't satiate and suppress hunger as well as solid food calories do. The upshot is that you're actually much more likely to overdrink a spinach, carrot, apple and caraway juice than you are to overeat a salad made from the same ingredients. Also, nutrients aren't the only things that are quickly and easily absorbed from juice. Even an 80 percent vegetable concoction will still be a concentrated source of natural sugars. This can have a rollercoaster effect on your blood sugar numbers, making your energy rapidly rise and just as quickly drop, especially if consumed on an empty stomach. So slip slow to get and keep that filling feeling.

THE BEST TIME TO POUR A REFILL

The rookie mistake is to drink too little. Actually, you want to be sipping about every two to three hours to feel full and keep your blood sugar levels on an even keel. Most cold press juice cleanses work on a regimen of around two cups of juice, usually four times a day; but if you feel you can't possibly sip another ounce after downing 35 ounces, then stop. Or if you've downed your 64-ounce portion and you're so hungry that you keep making Homer Simpson gurgling noises, then go ahead and have another (mostly green) juice—but thicken it with some fiber to stop your tummy rumbles (see "The Best Time to Bulk Up Your Cold Press Juice" on page 83 for high-fiber ingredient suggestions).

THE BEST TIME TO DRINK OTHER LIQUIDS

Drinking water and (decaffeinated) herbal tea while cleansing is needs-based. You don't want to overload if you aren't thirsty—too much liquid, known as water intoxication, can actually cause brain damage. The Mayo Clinic states that the adequate fluid intake is about 13 cups for men and about 9 cups for women. One to two liters of all liquids a day should be enough hydration (if you're getting enough, you'll pee every few hours and the urine will be on the clear side).

TIP All cleanses have an effect on your bowels. Since fiber intake is lower when cold press juicing, you're more likely to be backed up than letting loose with your movements. But whatever your intestinal reaction, water is the best cure. Diarrhea can cause dehydration, so you'll need to top up your body's liquid supply, while added fluids will help soften stool, making constipation easier to pass.

THE BEST TIME TO CUT OFF THE CALORIES

Surprise—since all the calories you're consuming are liquid, it's a slippery slope to drink over and under your daily limit. To lose a little weight but still have energy, count on at least 1,600 calories a day. If you consume fewer than 1,000 calories, your body will start acting like a figment of Stephen King's imagination, feeding on itself to conserve energy by burning muscle instead of fat. The calories in home-pressed juices are difficult to keep track of since you might need to add a little more of this or that to get the consistency you want and oranges vary from the size of a baseball to the size of a tennis ball. The recipes in this book generally weigh in under 200 calories each, unless they include nuts/nut butter (which are about 100 calories per tablespoon—protein does not come cheap) and most cold press liquids add up to between 100 and 350 calories per 16 ounces.

If you stick with a minimum of 80 percent veggies in your cold press juice cleanse, you're going to lose weight, no sweat. However, unless you have a plan in place for when you return to eating solids, you're probably going to regain that weight, no sweat. The purpose of a cleanse is to jump-start healthy eating intentions. So have a long-term post-cleanse eating plan in place. Continue to count calories (around 2,200 calories per day will keep you in skinny jeans) and pay attention to where those calories are coming from. Continue to eliminate processed foods and added sugars after your cleanse. Aim for five or six small meals a day, and focus on eating and occasionally drinking all of your RDA of fruit and veggies, including a serving or two of whole grains, healthy fat and lean protein.

THE BEST TIME TO BULK UP YOUR COLD PRESS JUICE

The midday juice. Skip adding some bulk to your snack-time juices and guaranteed, your get-happy-get-healthy cleanse will mutate into a trial of backed up, bone weary, bummed out misery. Most people don't get enough fiber (25 grams for women/38 grams for men) when they're not on a cleanse, let alone during a pure-produce cold press juice cleanse. Adding some extra fiber will also make you feel fuller and less likely to stray of the cleansing path due to cleansing hunger pangs.

Bulk up your juice with just four ounces of these ingredients:

○ Chia Seeds = 38 grams of fiber

○ Flaxseed = 27 grams of fiber

○ Wheat Germ = 13 grams of fiber

○ Almonds = 12 grams of fiber

○ Sunflower Seeds = 11 grams of fiber

○ Apples = 12 grams of fiber

TIP Mix the pulp into the finished drink.

THE BEST TIME TO WORK UP A SWEAT

After your first juice of the day. You'll be fueled and should generally have more get-up in your go first thing in the morning when cleansing. But opt for a warm, toasty feeling rather than going for your usual burn. Low on calories means high in fatigue, which can up your injury risk. Halve your usual routine or use this as the time to finally try yoga or Pilates, which are gently rigorous as opposed to muscle melt-down activities.

TIP Re-energize with another juice immediately after working out.

THE BEST TIME TO RE-CLEANSE IF YOU CHEATED

It happens. Don't beat yourself up with a wet asparagus stalk. Before cold pressing yourself back into your all-juice menu, figure out why you tripped up. It could be that this wasn't the right time—maybe you're just too busy/bleary-eyed/beat/befuddled/betwixt and between for a cleanse right now. After all, this isn't about living on liquids for a set period of time; you're overhauling your eating habits and developing a healthier lifestyle—not the sort of stuff that can be squeezed in between all of your other commitments. If it was more a matter of temptation than timing, dust yourself off and restart your cleanse ASAP, as if beginning from scratch, including easing out of your daily diet.

According to the *Annals of Behavioral Medicine*, there are four times when you're mostly likely to stray from your healthy-eating plans—knowledge is power and so is having a backup plan for the following all-too-likely scenarios:

#1 Snare—It's late at night

Snack time! Have an extra juice or, if you need something more, have the following no-cheat cheat foods on hand to see you through to the light of day (but be warned—eating solids in the middle of a cleanse can play a light fandango on your digestive system):

- ½ cup of pureed vegetables (make it something filling such as cucumbers, celery, avocado, broccoli or cauliflower; mashing it will make it easier on your digestive system)

- ¼ cup of unsalted, raw nuts

- 2 tablespoons of unsalted, 100 percent nut butter

- 8 ounces of low-sodium vegetable broth

- A green smoothie (it has similar nutritional stats to a green cold press juice, but the added fiber will satisfy your yen for something more substantial)

#2 Snare—You and your willpower are tired

In an ideal world, you would decamp to some tropical paradise while cleansing where you could while away the day drinking exotic produce out of a coconut shell, lying in a hammock and conjuring up happy Zen-like thoughts.

Unfortunately, you're more likely trying to fit your cleanse in between work, working out and keeping up with your friends, family and life in general. British researchers determined that keeping a cleansing journal will help you ID the life situations most likely to make you want to stray most. Try using one to create as ideal a world as possible in which to cleanse.

#3 Snare—There's booze on the premises

Go to the master. If anyone knows how to mix up a delicious all-juice cocktail, it's a bartender. Just hand over your mason jar and challenge them. You may end up with a few non-cleanse ingredients, but that's better than setting yourself up for a morning-after-the-night-before head-banger.

#4 Snare—You're hanging with friends

Your BFF may be great at giving you support, but you need someone who is experiencing the same pangs of hunger, moments of dizziness, frequent trips to the toilet, bouts of euphoria and flashes of determination that you're going through. Research published in the *Journal of Consulting and Clinical Psychology* established that people who buddy up are more likely to be successful when changing their eating habits than those who fly solo. But don't just fish on Craigslist for a cleansing chum—make sure the people you team up with have similar goals and aren't going to cave because it's TGIF (Thank Goodness It's Fried). Another option is to log on to one of the myriad of juicing sites and find yourself your own personal HJ who will cheerlead and harangue you, offer up recipes and tips, and generally Yoda you through your cleanse.

THE BEST TIME TO ADD PROTEIN

Protein helps build muscles, produce new cells, regulate hormones and enzymes, heal wounds and promote immune function. The Institute of Medicine recommends adults get a minimum of 0.8 grams of protein for every kilogram of body weight per day to keep from turning into some homemade horror flick in which the body slowly breaks down its own tissues to replenish its stores. That's just about 8 grams of protein for every 20 pounds of body weight. The best times to get that protein are early morning to replenish overnight stores, post–workout to feed tired muscles, between meals to prevent snacking urges and just before bed to tide you over until morning. But the bottom line is that at least one cold press juice a day should be beefed up with a dollop of the following high-protein foods:

○ Almonds

○ Amaranth

○ Asparagus

○ Broccoli

○ Buckwheat

○ Chia seeds

○ Cocoa powder

○ Hemp seeds

○ Peanuts

○ Quinoa

○ Sesame seeds

○ Spirulina

○ Sunflower seeds

THE BEST TIME TO START EATING SOLIDS

Just as you ease in to a cleanse, you also ease out. You probably won't be craving chips or pizza, but you may want to wrap your mouth around some protein-rich red meat or yogurt. Wait. Instead, take baby steps by chewing what you've been drinking—fruits and veggies, nuts and grains, but in whole form, with some light protein (eggs, fish, yogurt, tofu) thrown in. Spend at least half the number of days you cleansed to transition back to a more varied diet. After a couple of days, you can add healthy proteins like fish, poultry and lean meats, paying attention to how your body is reacting to each new bite. See "Clean Eating" on page 79 for a fuller menu of what post-cleanse ingredients to nix from your food world.

TIP Stick with small portions so as not to overwhelm your stomach and digestive system.

THE BEST TIME TO REFRAIN FROM CLEANSING

Cold press juice cleanses are not for everyone. The following are five instances when you absolutely should not cleanse.

1. You just finished a cleanse.

2. You are a woman who is pregnant or breastfeeding.

3. You have an autoimmune disease (drinking unpasteurized juices is dangerous).

4. You are on medication that you take with food (the cleanse can negatively interact with the prescription's efficacy).

5. You have a medical condition and didn't consult with your MD (particularly those with kidney disease, cancer, diabetes, heart disease or hypertension should consult with a medically licensed physician before embarking on any new eating/drinking plan).

THE BEST TIME TO DRINK COLD PRESS JUICE (OUTSIDE THE CLEANSE)

Since your cold press juice may be standing in as a liquid meal or snack, its ideal placement in your daily post-cleanse menu is important. The best time is on an empty belly either before or, if you prefer, in place of a snack or meal because many of the nutrients will be absorbed super quickly. If that seems too much to stomach, pair your cold press juice with protein. The research isn't conclusive, but the alkalinity in the juice may balance acid-producing foods like meat and cheese, which could protect against kidney stones, type 2 diabetes and colon cancer, strengthen bones and muscles, and improve heart health. The easiest time to gulp everything down is your first meal of the day (if you drink acid-producing coffee, make it an hour before or after your first cup).

THE BEST TIME TO POUR A REFILL (OUTSIDE THE CLEANSE)

Before eating, especially if you're trying to lose weight. Low-calorie, vegetable-laden juice just before your favorite meal can be just the ticket to shedding pounds. According to a Virginia Tech study, downing low-calorie liquid before every meal makes you feel fuller so you end up chowing down fewer calories. However, don't view this as an invitation to keep refilling your mason jar. If you aren't cleansing, stick to a strict two-drink or 200-calorie cold press juice maximum to keep your cold press juice a waistline-friendly part of your diet. While the disease-fighting potential of produce is considerable (read Chapter One again), vegetables and fruit move through your digestive system more quickly in juice form than they do in a whole state. So while a glass of juice might fill you up more in the short run, an *International Journal of Obesity* study found that when people were given either the solid or liquid version of certain foods (watermelon versus watermelon juice, cheese versus milk, and coconut meat versus coconut water), those who drank the liquids consumed up to 20 percent more calories throughout the rest of the day.

TIP Water down your cold press juice with ice, H2O, or club soda to pour on the amount you're drinking without piling on the calories.

NO EXCUSES—JUST JUICE IT

Overcome these 12 sometimes lame, sometimes legit excuses why today is not the day you will start your cleanse. (See "The Best Time to Refrain from Cleansing" on page 87 for the only truly justifiable times you should miss out on a cleanse.)

1. Legit: It looks like snow.

It's not your imagination—it's harder to start a cleanse when the mercury drops. Studies indicate that most people tend to eat more during the winter months, when the average person gains at least 1 to 2 pounds. The frostier temperatures, shorter days, longer nights and lack of sunshine collude to make us crave one thing: comfort food, which, unfortunately, tends to be high in everything but health. In addition, peak produce is in low supply, making it harder to work up an appetite for a cold press green juice.

Deal: Head to the freezer aisle for the freshest produce (see "Freeze Up" on page 48 for the fruits and vegetables that are always best bought on ice). Then spice your cold press juice with some heat—a dash of cayenne pepper, ginger, garlic or black pepper will warm you from within.

2. Lame: I have no time.

Deal: Yes, prepping for a cold press juice cleanse takes time. But you spent 62 hours binge-watching *Breaking Bad*. You spent 10 hours trying to progress to the next level in Candy Crush. You spent 10 minutes inhaling a wad of pizza dough hollowed out and stuffed with noodles, cream and cheese. You have the time.

3. Lame: I am So. Tired. Of. Juice.

Deal: There are an estimated 2,000 edible fruit and vegetables in the world. That adds up to a lot of different variations of juice. Experiment. You'll get it wrong occasionally, but it's more fun than just limiting yourself to the same 10 ingredients. Flip to Section II for some ideas to get you cold pressing.

4. Lame: I'm not getting anything done because I have to pee every 20 minutes.

Deal: It takes less than a minute to pee and another to (hopefully) wash your hands. Two minutes, even every 20 minutes, only adds up to six minutes an hour—about the time it takes to update your FB page.

5. Legit: I am soooooooooooooo tired.

Of course you're feeling like you need a nap. It's not just the upshot of eating fewer calories. You're also stimulant deprived—sugar, caffeine, alcohol and nicotine are often go-tos for getting through the day.

Deal: This is why the best time to start a cleanse is on a weekend or when you have downtime so you can flake out and nap during the day. If you really need a boot to the pants, opt for a midday cold press with a medium- to high-sugar fruit.

Medium-High Sugar Content	High Sugar Content
Plums	Tangerines
Oranges	Cherries
Kiwis	Grapes
Pears	Mangos
Pineapples	

6. Legit: I feel like I just spent the day on a roller coaster.

The change in diet and reduction in calories might make you feel dizzy or a little nauseous initially.

Deal: Don't soldier through it—your stomach is telling you it needs to be fed. Listen to it. Part of a successful cleanse is getting in tune with what your body needs. To get through the spacey light-headed phase, add a spoonful of protein to your juicer; nuts or seeds will satisfy your cravings without sacrificing your cleanse.

7. Legit: I'm starving.

Deal: Same MO as dealing with dizziness and nausea. Pack some protein into your presser (say that five times fast to test your cognitive reactions).

8. Lame: I miss chewing.

Deal: Actually, some Hardcore Juicers recommend that you chew your green juice. There is solid science to back up the wisdom of masticating a liquid: A Purdue University study found that digestion begins in the mouth and food that is broken down as much as possible—even juice—helps the body retain more nutrients than poorly chewed food.

9. Legit: Juicing is crazy expensive.

Granted, shelling out cash for a juicer will leave a hole in your bank account. And produce—fresh or frozen—can be more expensive than processed food.

Deal: Now think about what you spend for a coffee or a bottle of water on a daily basis. Add in how expensive a heart attack, type 2 diabetes, cancer and the myriad of other serious health conditions associated with not getting your daily nine will be. You can afford the occasional cleanse.

10. Legit: There is no hard evidence that drinking vegetables and fruits is better for you than eating them.

Deal: True. But unless you plan on mainlining kale, there is no easier way to eat your weight in produce, which is essentially what the RDA seems to equal.

11. Legit: I hate cleansing alone.

Research in the *Journal of Consulting and Clinical Psychology* confirms that any dietary change is more likely to be successful when you buddy up.

Deal: Find a juicing pal, but put as much thought into what you want from your cleansing chum as you did picking out your juicer. For instance:

○ Do you want someone who will hold hands and sympathize with you or someone who will hold you accountable for every vegetable you cold press?

○ Do you want a virtual or actual support group?

○ Does it matter if you have similar schedules?

○ Do you want to be like the faceless person icon on FB or get up close and personal?

12. Lame: Everyone's going out for drinks.

Deal: One word: thermos. Bring your green drink with you. So you end up being the designated driver. Think of all the stories you can make up about who did what with whom! Or ask the bartender to flex their mixologist skills and wow you with an all-juice, green cocktail.

THE BEST TIME TO LET THE WORLD KNOW THAT YOU'RE ON A CLEANSE

Before you start. This way, you won't have to listen to objections (try my all-candy cleanse!), negative comments (cleanses are for people who have no willpower), snide remarks (Mars called and they're short one green martian) and rah-rah cheerleading from someone who doesn't understand what the cleanse entails (it's almost nighttime so you can have a cocktail). Earlier also means you're giving everyone the heads-up that it's better to give you a wide berth when you're in the midst of cleansing and self-focused to the point where you think your spouse's best friend or your boss will really want to hear about your bowels or how sharp your focus is or the exact size you need to cut a carrot to easily push it through the juicer.

THE BEST TIME TO CLEANSE FOR HEALTH

Unlike your car, your body does not come with an owner's manual telling you how often to take it in for a service. But your system can use a regular tune-up and, in fact, a regular clean-out of your lungs and gastrointestinal tract (in layman terms, the systems that filter the junk out of your body) can optimize your protection against a *Merck Manual* of medical conditions. A three-to-seven day cold press juice cleanse every three months can help keep your engine clog-free and running smoothly. Juicing up on certain fruits and vegetables will help extend the life of your machine and it's individual parts:

Arteries

Cholesterol can turn your arteries into an LA highway during rush hour.

JUICING PREVENTATIVE CARE: Pears, grapes, cranberries, citrus fruit, cucumbers and apples all contain antioxidants that can help ward off damage caused by free radicals, like plaque buildup and high LDL cholesterol levels.

Liver

The Swiss Army knife of the organs, the liver has around 250 functions. The three big ones are filtering the bacteria and pollutants in your body by cleaning blood, producing bile (the digestive goo that helps the body process fat) and storing the sugar glycogen (your body's go-to backup fuel when it needs some instant get-up-and-go).

JUICING PREVENTATIVE CARE: Folate, or vitamin B9, helps keep the liver multitasking like a well-oiled tool. Rich sources include beets, parsley, asparagus, broccoli and spinach.

TIP Avoid grapefruits when taking prescription (or over-the-counter) medications, as it interacts with liver enzymes in a way that can keep the medication in your system longer than expected.

Bones

Without a cache of calcium, vitamin D, magnesium and phosphorus, bones are in danger of losing their density.

JUICING PREVENTATIVE CARE: Broccoli is one of the few veggies high in calcium, while kiwi, parsley, tomatoes and kale are good sources of vitamin K, which aids in the absorption of calcium and, therefore, overall bone health.

TIP Skip spinach for bone-building. Although it's strong in calcium, it also contains oxalic acid, which can interfere with the body's absorption of the calcium.

Guts

The guts, or gastrointestinal tract, which runs from your esophagus down into your stomach, small intestine and colon, works like a 24/7 traffic cop, separating and directing the protein, carbohydrates, fat, vitamins and minerals for body lock-up or release. Anything that interferes and obstructs this system's functioning can prevent your body from soaking up nutrients and cause attacks of heartburn, bloating and abdominal pain.

JUICING PREVENTATIVE CARE: The GI tract needs to be roughed up to prevent blockages. Since even cold press juice is fiber-challenged, choose produce that gives the most stool bang for its bulk, such as leafy greens (especially kale and spinach), green beans, raspberries, cherries, sweet potatoes, nut milks, oat milk and the skins as well as the "meat" of cucumbers, apples and pears.

Brain

Research has established that the brain regenerates in the same way as any other organ and keeps making new neurons.

JUICING PREVENTATIVE CARE: Look for ingredients with antioxidants that boost cognitive function by increasing blood flow to the brain. Beets, blueberries, blackberries and coconut water all keep your brain cells firing efficiently.

Lungs

While the lungs have their own self-cleaning cycle, smog, smoke, pollution and whatever other gunk is airborne in your breathing vicinity can all clog up the works and cause inflammation.

JUICING PREVENTATIVE CARE: It sounds like something Dr. Leo Spaceman would say, but it's true that food can help your breathe better. Produce high in retinoic acid, or vitamin A (think orange/yellow fruit and vegetables), helps your lungs rebuild while the pectin and antioxidants in apples and their peels have been shown to reduce inflammation.

Kidneys

These organs work like your own personal sewage water treatment plant, except instead of filtering H2O, they cleanse the blood of around two quarts of excess water daily, waste and by-products of digestion. This helps regulate blood pressure and keep the heart happy, so you want to make sure the kidneys aren't struggling to balance out the fluids in your body.

JUICING PREVENTATIVE CARE: Coming up dry can cause the kidneys to shut down, so any juice with liquid added will keep things swimming along. Adding some oranges will boost the flow and help prevent kidney stones from forming.

JUICING SOLUTIONS

Cleanse your medicine cabinet with these cold press juice ingredient prescriptions for whatever ails you.

TAKE 10 YEARS OFF: Ditch the expensive skin creams. Cucumbers are hydrating and rich in minerals such as potassium, magnesium and silica, which are believed to even out skin tone and add a healthy, vibrant glow.

STOP FEELING MORE RUN-DOWN THAN A CHEVROLET VEGA: Orange, strawberry and grapefruit are vitamin C powerhouses that can help boost your immune system and fight off viruses.

FEEL AS BRIGHT-EYED AS A BUNNY: Kiwis and blackberries contain vitamins A, C and E, which all play a role in keeping our eyes sharp.

LEAP TALL BUILDINGS IN A SINGLE BOUND: You need nuts (protein) and spinach (potassium) for muscle repair, plus red cabbage (antioxidant plant compound anthocyanin) and ground flaxseed (omega-3 fats) to reduce inflammation.

BE PICTURE-READY: If you have a bruise, load up on vitamin C (citrus) to shore up blood vessels, vitamin K (kale) to reduce blood clotting and vitamin E (broccoli) to reap the benefits of cytokines (a molecule that mimics over-the-counter anti-inflammatory medications).

GET FASTER, STRONGER, LEANER: Beets have been shown to help the body convert nitrates into nitric acid, a gas that widens blood vessels. Bottom line: You'll significantly improve your workout performance.

GET ALL THE WINK, WINK, NUDGE, NUDGE BENEFITS OF DOWNING A BUCKETFUL OF CHOCOLATE AND OYSTERS, WITHOUT THE CHOLESTEROL OR CALORIES: Celery contains androsterone, a male hormone that acts as a come-hither pheromone (plus it freshens breath, which sweetens the action post-hithering) while asparagus is high in vitamin E, which is known as the "sex vitamin" because it pretty much slam dunks everything "lurve," from boosting attraction, desire and mood to cranking out sex hormones to aiding in lubrication.

GET MOVING AND GROOVING: Skip the triple espresso and add some chlorophyll to your juice. The extra punch of green pigment helps oxygenate the blood, creating increased brain function and energy.

SATISFY YOUR SUGAR CRAVINGS: Beets and carrots have a sweet edge while cinnamon contains compounds that help stabilize blood sugar and therefore minimize your sugar jones.

NEVER FEEL EMBARRASSED IN PUBLIC AGAIN: Adding ginger to juice helps relax the intestinal tract and reduce gas. Lemon and mint are also tummy tamers.

STOP THE ACHES AND PAINS OF COLD AND FLU BEFORE THEY START: Try an antioxidant boilermaker of vitamin A (apricots, cabbage, cantaloupe, carrots, collard greens, grapefruit, Romaine lettuce, mango, pepper, spinach, sweet potato, tomato and watermelon) to bolster your immunity and overall mucous membrane health; vitamin C (berries, broccoli, Brussels sprouts, cantaloupe, cauliflower, grapefruit, honeydew, kale, kiwi, mango, nectarine, orange, sweet potato, strawberries, tomatoes and red, green or yellow peppers) to stop a cold short in its tracks; and vitamin E (broccoli, carrots, chard, mustard greens, mangos, nuts, red peppers, spinach and sunflower seeds) to double-whammy your immune defenses; and with a shot of zinc (endive, alfalfa sprouts, squashes, zucchini, broccoli rabe, spinach, asparagus, parsley and radicchio) to speed recovery.

CHAPTER FIVE
COMING CLEAN

A juice cleanse isn't a one-size-fits-all program. Depending on your needs and your cleansing hacker skills, it can be as short as a 24-hour blast, continue for a few days, or, for those with some cleansing experience under their belt and in their tummies, last as long as a week. Refresh the cleansing basics in the previous chapter if you need to and then choose your plan.

THE FIVE STAGES OF CLEANSING

No matter how long you cleanse, your mental state will pass through some variation of the following:

STAGE ONE: THIS ISN'T THAT BAD

I can totally do this. I'll get to chopping early before work, I'll add some cinnamon and cacao nibs, I love kale, I'll do a long workout this afternoon. I'll bet this will be a breeze. I'm good!

This is your happy place. A feeling of euphoria—something like a runner's high—gets triggered in the first flush of a cleanse as you begin to feel a triumph over your impulse-control issues. Remember it and use it as your reference point when your mind hits Stages Two through Four.

STAGE TWO: "HANGER," OR WHAT HAPPENS WHEN "HUNGER" MEETS "ANGER"

Panic! Panic! Everything smells like food, even my pet dog/cat/fish. Everyone seems to be eating. The world is turning into walking versions of those mutant turkey legs you get at Disneyland. I hate everyone. Help me! I'm starving.

Your body is entering fight-or-flight (or, in this case, fight-or-feed) survival mode. The sudden drop in calories can send a shock to your system, which manifests as extreme hunger. To get through Stage Two, try adding some nut butter to your next cold press. It'll bulk up your drink and make you feel fuller longer.

STAGE THREE: BARGAINING

Okay, breathe. I feel totally F'd (famished/fed up/flaky/fragile/foggy/frantic/farty and full of s*&t). Maybe I'll just take a little break. A cup of coffee won't kill me (see "Get Your Java Jolt" on page 98). Would it be so terrible if I eat an apple instead of juice it?

The cut in calories leads to blood sugar levels dropping, while the lack of carbs forces your body to switch to feeding off of tiny fat cells known as ketones, making you feel like you just slugged out few rounds with Mike Tyson. You're tired, headachy and completely out of sorts. The good news is that ketones are your brain's preferred food, so ride this out and you'll get back to that Stage One ode to joy. The better news is that ketones reduce hunger so your friends will no longer look delicious. To help get you through the brain fog without screwing up at work or in your life, boost cognitive thinking by throwing some omega-3 fatty acid–rich ingredients like ground flaxseed, walnuts and chia seeds into your daily cold pressing.

A Harvard University–led study has determined that switching diets also freaks the microbiome (aka gut bug population) which causes that not-so-sweet backlash in your intestinal functioning. The result: You'll get to know various bathroom décor in your world very, very well. While these symptoms are part and parcel of any cleanse, you can minimize the tummy troubles by including one kombucha-based juice daily. According to the *World Journal of Gastroenterology*, fermented foods can ease gastric distress.

STAGE FOUR: DOUBT

I'm never going to make this. I am the world's worst cleanser. Bad! Bad! I hate myself.

One of the hardest parts of a cleanse actually isn't the restricted diet—it's having to rethink your social life so that all of your eating and drinking moments revolve around things that come out of a juicer (mojitos don't count unless they're the faux green version on page 162). When you're down and troubled and you need a helping hand, you need a friend. Folk singer James Taylor, the purple dinosaur Barney, the old game show *Who Wants to Be a Millionaire* and any TV sitcom ensemble all know the value of friends. This is the time to gather your cleansing peeps and get some words of encouragement. Then hit the toilet.

STAGE FIVE: SUCCESS

Epiphany moment: I feel great. I look great. I am great. I can climb Everest. Okay, maybe not—but I can definitely destroy a few flights of stairs. It doesn't even bother me that someone is eating waffles and bacon within my sniffing vicinity. I can totally do this. In fact, I can do this forever. I will do this forever. Juicing is my new life.

Once your body has adapted to its new restricted diet, the good times flow. However, for the reasons mentioned above, never extend a cleanse beyond its expiration date. If you're on a one-day cleanse, then that is what you stick to, and so on. You chose the specific program for a reason. This isn't to say you should stick to solids except when cleansing—go ahead and substitute a fresh green drink for a daily meal. The point is that juicing is a way of life; cleansing is a way to get into that life.

GET YOUR JAVA JOLT

If you can't make it a morning, let alone a week, without your daily perk, these mock mochas have just enough kick to get you moving without the caffeine jitters.

BEECHNUTS: Remove from husk and roast until dark and brittle. Grind and brew like coffee, using 1 teaspoon per cup of water (beware of squirrels when drinking).

CHICORY ROOT: These blue flowers with almost leafless stalks grow just about everywhere there's a road (preferably harvest in an unsprayed area). They look like daisies, but their petals are blue and squared off at the ends. Roast the white fleshy roots until dark brown and brittle, then grind and prepare like coffee, using ½ tablespoon per cup of water.

DANDELION ROOT: Follow the same instructions as for chicory root (preferably harvest in an unsprayed area).

PARSNIPS: Finely chop (or grate) a batch of fresh parsnip roots (skins and all) to the consistency of hashbrown potatoes. Dehydrate (if using the oven, at 150°F for around 10 hours and then roast them at 400°F for about 20 minutes until they're a very dark brown). Steep 1 rounded tablespoon per cup of scalding hot water.

WHEAT: Mix 6 cups of ground or cracked wheat with 1 cup of water, ½ cup of molasses and ½ teaspoon of ground celery seeds to a pasty consistency, spread on lined cookie sheets and bake at 350°F until toasty brown (keep an eye on it for the last 10 minutes, as it easily burns). Turn the oven off and let the paste cool (it should be crisp). Grind. Brew 1½ tablespoons per cup of hot water.

CHICKPEAS: Roast in a 300°F oven for about 45 minutes until they turn the color of roasted coffee beans. Grind and use 1 tablespoon per cup of water (this coffee sub works best in a percolator or boiled and strained rather than in a drip coffee maker).

UNHULLED BARLEY: Dry-toast in heavy pan over medium heat for 10 minutes, stirring occasionally, until completely dark brown. Grind and use 1 heaping teaspoon per cup of water.

MEAL PLANS: WHAT TO EAT BEFORE AND AFTER CLEANSING

The single word that stands between success and frustration when cleansing is "preparation." This goes for your daily menu plan as well. Cleaning up what you put in your body before diving into a cleanse will get you ready mentally and physically for an all-juice diet. The ideal is to prepare for at least half as long as you are going to cleanse—so half day before a one-day cleanse, one-

and-a-half days before a three-day cleanse and two-and-a-half days before a five-day cleanse, start choosing your meals from the healthy low-fat, high-protein, 100 percent filling suggestions below (add two snacks/desserts as needed). Use spices as desired and drink from the beverages listed in "Liquid Diet" (page 103).

BREAKFASTS

QUICK BITE: Mix ½ cup plain yogurt with 1 tablespoon chopped almonds and ½ grapefruit on the side.

HEARTY START: Top ½ cup your choice of grain with ½ cup your choice of chopped fruit and 1 teaspoon cinnamon.

TOFU VEGGIE SCRAMBLE: Chop extra-firm tofu in bite-size pieces and sauté 10 minutes in a pan lightly coated with olive oil over medium high heat. When the tofu is dry and slightly crispy, add 2 chopped tomatoes and your choice of ¼ cup chopped fresh herbs. Cook 5 more minutes, stirring.

NO-GUILT EGGS BENEDICT: Poach 1 egg and serve over 1 brown rice cake topped with ¼ ounce grated strong-flavored cheese such as cheddar or Parmesan.

DINER DELIGHT: Mix ½ cup your choice of cooked grain with ½ cup chopped peaches.

FREEDOM OMELET: Cut ½ cup your choice of vegetables in thin slices and sauté for 2 minutes over medium-high heat in a small pan. Set aside. Beat 1 egg with 1 tablespoon of water and cook in the same pan over medium-low heat for 2 minutes. When eggs begin to set, gently lift edges with a spatula and tilt the pan so the uncooked part of the egg flows toward the edges. After 2 more minutes, when egg looks dry, spoon the veggies in the center and gently fold one edge of the omelet over them. Cook 1 more minute.

MONKEY SMOOTHIE: Chop 2 medium bananas, 1 apple and 2 cups spinach and blend with ½ cup orange juice, ½ cup water and 1 tablespoon ground flaxseed to make a 16-ounce drink.

LUNCHES

BUTTERBALL BOWL: Chop and mix 2 ounces lean turkey breast, 1 ounce mozzarella cheese and ½ cup your choice of vegetables. Add 15 halved grapes and drizzle with no more than 1 teaspoon fruity vinegar such as strawberry or raspberry.

CUP O' LENTIL: Sprinkle 1 tablespoon feta cheese over 2 cups hot lentil soup.

THE WHOLE GRAIN SALAD: Mix your choice of ½ cup cooked grains with 1 small chopped tomato, 1 cup diced zucchini and 2 sliced green onions, and drizzle with 2 teaspoons lemon juice mixed with 1 teaspoon olive oil.

TUNA SALAD NICOISE: Mix 3 cups salad greens with 3 ounces water-packed albacore white tuna, 1 small sliced tomato, 3 red onion slices, ½ cup green beans and ½ medium chopped cucumber. Drizzle with 1 teaspoon olive oil mixed with 2 tablespoons rice vinegar and crumble ¼ cup brown rice cakes on top.

YOGURT CUP: Mix 6 ounces plain Greek-style yogurt with 1 cup of your choice of chopped fruit.

CHIC SALAD: Place 2½ ounces lean grilled chicken (skin removed) on top of 2 cups salad greens. Drizzle with 1 tablespoon of olive oil. Grate ½ ounce Parmesan cheese on top. Serve with 5 rice or millet crackers on the side.

SPINACH SALAD: Mix 1 cup torn spinach leaves with 14 walnut halves, ½ cup broccoli, 1 ounce crumbled feta and ⅓ cup dried cranberries, and drizzle with 1 tablespoon balsamic vinegar.

DINNERS

SALAD BAR: Mix 1 tablespoon hummus with ½ cup shredded carrots and ¼ cup sprouts. Serve on a plate with 2 ounces roasted chicken breast (skin removed), ¼ cup rice or your choice of cooked grains and ½ cup shredded Romaine lettuce mixed with ½ cup avocado.

BIG BOWL CHOPPED SALAD: Chop 3 ounces salmon, ½ cup broccoli, ½ cauliflower and ½ cucumber in bite-size pieces, and mix in a bowl with 1 tablespoon your choice of chopped nuts, ½ cup brown rice and 1 tablespoon miso paste or 1 teaspoon miso powder.

FISHY DINNER: Squeeze ½ lemon over 3 ounces baked trout and serve with ¼ cup wild rice and ½ cup roasted tomatoes mixed with ½ cup steamed kale and ¼ cup cooked chickpeas.

ASIAN STIR-FRY: Sauté ½ cup tofu in 1 tablespoon sesame oil with garlic and ginger over medium-high heat until spices are browned. Add 1 cup sliced bok choy, ½ cup snow peas and 1 cup sliced mushrooms and stir-fry for 2 more minutes. Add ½ cup cooked brown rice and cook, stirring, for 2 minutes before serving.

MUSHROOM BURGER: Marinate 1 large portobello mushroom cap in 1 tablespoon balsamic vinegar for 20 minutes. Broil/grill on high close to heat for 3 to 5 minutes per side (until slightly crispy). Serve with lettuce, tomato, onions and 1 tablespoon mustard on a gluten-free bun with 8 spears of broiled/grilled asparagus and ½ cup broiled/grilled cubed squash on the side.

MEDITERRANEAN STIR-FRY: Sauté 3 ounces firm tofu, 1 chopped tomato, 1 cup chopped spinach, 1 cup summer squash, tomatoes, eggplant and/or onion in 1 tablespoon olive oil over medium-high heat. Sprinkle with 1 tablespoon feta before serving.

SUSHI PLATE: Mix 1 tablespoon miso paste with 1 teaspoon water and brush over ½ cup tofu. Broil under high heat until crispy. Serve with 8 pieces brown rice vegetable sushi and ½ cup seaweed salad.

SNACKS/DESSERTS

NUTTY STICKS: Spread 1 tablespoon 100 percent nut butter on 6 celery sticks.

FRUIT SALAD: 1 cup your choice chopped fruit.

JAPANESE SNACK: ½ cup cooked edamame, served warm.

GREEN JUICE: Choose any recipe from this book.

CHOCOLATE FRO-FRUIT: Puree your choice of 1 cup fruit, mix with 1 tablespoon unsweetened cocoa and freeze in an ice tray or a small cup with a stick to make an ice pop.

SALSA AND VEGGIE CHIPS: Mix ¼ cup black beans with 1 tablespoon salsa, 1 tablespoon plain yogurt and ¼ cup mashed avocado and serve with 4 celery stalks.

FRO-FRUIT ENCORE: Freeze 15 grapes or berries.

NUT BAR: Roll ½ banana in 1 tablespoon cacao nibs.

LIQUID DIET

The following thirst-quenchers can be swigged as needed throughout your cleansing day:

WATER/SELTZER: Although uncommon, it's possible to drink too much water (see "The Best Time to Drink Other Liquids" on page 81).

FLAVORED WATER/SELTZER: Lightly mash fruits/herbs/spices/vegetables in a glass and add water/seltzer. Mint, ginger, melons, cucumbers, citrus and berries are tasty options.

HERBAL TEAS: Pour 1 pint of boiling water over 1 ounce of fresh or dried herbs and steep, or, if using seeds or roots, simmer for 10 to 60 minutes (depending on how flavor-intense you like it). Strain. Add ice if drinking cold.

CLEANSE 1: ONE-DAY QUICKIE CLEANSING PLAN

If you can barely get through the next hour, let alone the day, without multiple coffees, Red Bull, candy and electronic cigarettes, if you wake up every morning with a puffy, pimply sugar face and as pale as a cast member of *True Blood*, if you ate and drank your way through the weekend and now feel fatter than Albert and more run-down than a two-year-old cell phone, you need to cleanse. And you need to do it fast. The One-Day Quickie cleanse will get and keep you on a healthy life track. It may only last 24 hours, but it is a lifetime plan. You're giving yourself the opportunity to take a breath and reassess your lifestyle.

The beauty of a quickie is that it needs no prep (though a little Boy Scout mentality never goes amiss) and not only can you do it as often as you like, new research suggests you should be doing it every few days. A study published in the *International Journal of Obesity* suggests consuming fewer than 1,200 calories three to four days a week and the average 2,000 (women) to 2,400 (men) calories needed daily to maintain weight the rest of the time is as or more effective than reducing one's calories to between 1,200 and 1,500 calories daily. In addition to dropping pounds, the reported health effects of this kind of intermittent fasting reads like a laundry list of Vulcan-like live-long-and-prosper benefits including: a reduction in cardiovascular risk markers such as lowered triglycerides and cholesterol numbers, improved blood pressure, slowed cancer cell growth, higher production of the hormones responsible for the breakdown of lipids, better blood sugar and appetite control, increased fat burning and metabolic rate, stronger cognitive skills and higher cell turnover and repair.

Also in the gain column is the fact that this kind of short-burst cleansing schedule is easy to start and stick to, especially once it becomes an old habit (if it's Tuesday, it must be cleanse day). However, it takes about two weeks of regular intermittent fasting for your body to adjust, so expect some room-clearing gastrointestinal pushback initially.

TIP Don't hang out with non-cleansing friends during even a quickie juice cleanse because receiving a text inviting you to "lattes at *" will definitely make you irrationally angry.

Quickie cleanses are usually initiated after a stint of living like a before picture of a *The Biggest Loser* applicant, so no assembly is required once you gather your ingredients. However, if the down-the-road plan is to interval cleanse on a weekly basis, then thinking ahead and thinning out your diet can only step up the long-term health gains and weight loss. So at least a day before cleansing, choose a dish from each meal in the "Meal Plans: What to Eat Before and After Cleansing" section (page 99) and phase out the unhealthy food items listed in "Clean Eating" (page 79).

RAINBOW JUICE SAMPLE MENU

While 80 percent green vegetable drinks are the backbone of a healthy cold press juice cleanse, for the newbie juicer, starting cold turkey with just greens and nothing but greens can bring back bad memories of your mother telling you to eat your vegetables. Drinking a rainbow not only gradually shifts you into all-verdant territory, the color scheme makes it easy to remember (just memorize the name Roy G. Biv for Red, Orange, Yellow, Green, Blue, Indigo, Violet) and varied enough to keep your taste buds thirsty.

RED

- Cherry Pop (page 134)
- Strawberry Milkshake (page 136)

ORANGE

- Creamsicle (page 145)
- What's Up Doc? (page 140)

YELLOW

- Curry Chai (page 155)
- Lemonade (page 155)

GREEN

- Beach Bum (page 161)
- Sweet Greens (page 138)

BLUE

- Blue Blood (page 162)
- Blue Moon (page 159)

INDIGO

- Mood Indigo (page 172)
- Smurf Juice (page 176)

VIOLET

- Purple Cow (page 146)
- Purple Power (page 183)

MONO JUICE MENU

For the experienced juicers, pick one all-vegetable drink and make this the foundation of your cleanse. The reason the mono plan is more for those who have already drunk the green Kool-Aid and have some cleansing know-how is that it takes a little more effort (i.e., the ability to ignore your gag reflex) to drink the same liquid salad for breakfast, lunch, dinner and all of your snacks. The reason you want to keep the ingredients exclusive is that it's a fast way to overhaul your diet. Eating the same thing morning, noon and night means that you're less likely to use food to fill other voids in your life so you'll therefore consume fewer and healthier calories. Scientists call this the "habituation" effect—the body's decreasing response to a stimulus after repeated exposure to it—and say it's a useful tool for shedding weight.

- In the Green (page 128)

- Green Goddess (page 128)

- Green Acres (page 129)

- Green-Eyed Monster (page 129)

PRACTICALS

○ Drink from the Liquid Diet (page 103) as needed (listen to your body and sip when you're thirsty).

○ Plan on drinking a total of 64 ounces of fresh cold press juice.

○ The general rule of thumb is to aim to drink 8 ounces of juice every two hours.

○ Block out a down day when you can kick back and relax.

○ Finish the last juice two hours before you sleep.

○ Start your cleanse 12 hours before your morning wake-up call; so, if your alarm is set for 8 a.m., stop eating at 8 p.m. the night before. Good news; by the time you wake up, you're already a third of the way into your cleanse!

Newbie Timetable

Wake-Up Time	8 ounces any drink from the Liquid Diet list (page 103)
Breakfast of Champions (30 minutes later)	8 ounces of a red cold press juice
Snack (2 hours later)	8 ounces of an orange cold press juice
Liquid Lunch (2 hours later)	8 ounces of a yellow cold press juice
Afternoon Sugar Craving (2 hours later)	8 ounces of a green cold press juice
Happy Hour (2 hours later)	8 ounces of a blue cold press juice
Not-the-Dog's Dinner (2 hours later)	8 ounces of an indigo cold press juice
Sweet Course (2 hours later)	8 ounces of a violet cold press juice
Late-Night Munchies (2 hours later)	8 ounces of color of your choice cold press juice
To Get You through the Night	8 ounces any drink from the Liquid Diet list (page 103)

Hardcore Timetable

Wake-Up Time	8 ounces any drink from the Liquid Diet list (page 103)
Breakfast of Champions (30 minutes later)	8 ounces of your chosen Mono Juice
Snack (2 hours later)	8 ounces of your chosen Mono Juice
Liquid Lunch (2 hours later)	8 ounces of your chosen Mono Juice
Afternoon Sugar Craving (2 hours later)	8 ounces of your chosen Mono Juice
Happy Hour (2 hours later)	8 ounces of your chosen Mono Juice
Not-the-Dog's Dinner (2 hours later)	8 ounces of your chosen Mono Juice
Sweet Course (2 hours later)	8 ounces of your chosen Mono Juice
Late-Night Munchies (2 hours later)	8 ounces of your chosen Mono Juice
To Get You through the Night	8 ounces any drink from the Liquid Diet list (page 103)

TIP Throw the pulp back into your juice at lunch to add midday fiber and/ or bulk up your morning or snack juice up with some protein (see "The Best Time to Add Protein" on page 85).

BACK TO REAL LIFE

Don't just jump back into the feeding trough the morning after your cleanse. Instead of being ruled by an "it's breakfast, so it's time to eat" mentality, wait until your body has its "feed me, Seymour" moment. Your post-cleanse cleanup menu will be identical to your pre-cleanse one; for at least one day following your cleanse, choose a dish from each meal in "Meal Plans: What to Eat Before and After Cleansing" (page 99). Try to choose dairy- and wheat-free meals the first day. Pay attention to how your body reacts with each new ingredient. But whether you reboot in a week or plan for a lengthier cleanse next time, continue to shut the pantry door on the unhealthy ingredients listed in "Clean Eating" (page 79) from your daily menu.

CLEANSE 2: THE THREE-DAY KICK-BUTT, BELLY-BUSTING, EAT-LESS-CRAP CLEANSE

You need to drop some ballast and you need to drop it right now. This cleanse will do it. It's tough to maintain, especially if you haven't cleansed before, but it's just short enough for you to be able to drink your way through it and just long enough to do the job. Follow the menu plan and you'll lose, on average, three to eight pounds, guaranteed.

But before you dash off and invest in a new, sized-down wardrobe, know that the wake-up-and-smell-the-chocolate reality is that there are no quick fixes when it comes to keeping that weight off. So while 72 hours of only drinking cold press juice may be enough to blast you through your big event, the long-term purpose of this cleanse is to have a healthier chow routine once you start eating whole foods again. When you're creating new dietary habits, it's best to start with a win. Danish researchers found that losing big early in a diet makes for more successful weight loss in the long-term by putting a fire in your belly and boosting your backbone when it comes to passing on your trigger foods. You might still regain some of the weight (since a portion of the loss is water), but your three days of making your daily diet the focus of your life means that you'll be more aware of what you're putting in your mouth. This mindful eating can help minimize the kind of indulgent, "I need a bacon burger and I need it now" rebound appetite that a multitude of studies have determined is one of the leading culprits to regained weight after any restricted food program.

It also means you can wave buh-bye to calorie counting. When you relearn food in the context of your individual body and its needs, you'll load your fork with healthy, nutritional choices that are right for you, that fill you up and don't leave you craving a pint of Moose Tracks ice cream at 3 a.m.

Before you start the three-day cleanse, cut the crap. Seriously. No more:

C Carbonated Drinks, Candy, Caffeine, Carbohydrates (gluten), Cheese (and other full-fat dairy foods) and Cigarettes

R Refined sugar and Red meat

A Artificial sweeteners/colors and Alcohol

P Processed foods and Preservatives

At least 36 hours before starting a three-day cleanse, your diet should be cleaner than Madonna's colon. The simplest guideline: If this is something that would make it into an Elvis Presley cookbook, then you probably shouldn't be eating it as cleanse prep. The even simpler guideline: Choose a dish from each meal in "Meal Plans: What to Eat Before and After Cleansing" (page 99).

TIP To keep your taste buds from staging an intervention before you even begin your cleanse, spike your food and water with lots of strong spices and flavorings such as cinnamon, cayenne, turmeric, curry, hot pepper flakes, garlic, ginger, mint and paprika.

The three-day cleanse is for newcomers and experienced cleansers alike, although the biggest challenge for those who haven't lived on what is essentially liquid salad for multiple days will be the four vegetable to one fruit ratio. If you're having trouble stomaching it, rather than rework the numbers (which can have a backlash effect on your own measurements), throw in an occasional extra carrot, sweet potato or beet. It'll sweeten the deal without jacking up fructose levels.

THREE-DAY CLEANSE SAMPLE MENU

Choose one of the suggested juices below for each meal during your Three-Day cleanse—you can try all three over the course of your cleanse or stick with a favorite:

BREAKFAST OF CHAMPIONS
- "Green Tea" (page 131)
- Kick Start (page 131)
- Sunrise Surprise (page 133)

SNACK
- Gingerbread (page 140)
- Goin' Nutz (page 148)
- Trail Mix (page 141)

LIQUID LUNCH
- Big Three (page 151)
- Chef Salad (page 151)
- Twilight (page 156)

AFTERNOON SUGAR CRAVING
- Chocolate Silk (page 143)
- Peanut Butter Cup (page 138)
- Sweet Potato Pie (page 143)

HAPPY HOUR
- Hawaiian Punch (page 158)
- Kick-Ass Lemonade (page 158)
- Pink Drink (page 159)

NOT-THE-DOG'S DINNER
- Kissing a Cow (page 167)
- Spicy Mexican Green (page 152)

- Sweet and Sour (page 167)

SWEET COURSE
- Cherry Pie (page 177)
- Neapolitan (page 173)
- Tropical Delight (page 176)

LATE-NIGHT MUNCHIES
- Happy Dreams (page 181)
- Hot Cocoa (page 184)
- Vanilla Chai (page 185)

TIP Don't live in fat fear; the omega-3 fats found in nuts and seeds help produce the blubber-burning enzyme PPAR-alpha, which also slows down fat storage and helps keep you full and in control of your appetite.

PRACTICALS

○ Drink from the Liquid Diet (page 103) as needed (listen to your body and sip when you're thirsty).

○ Plan on drinking 8 ounces of fresh cold press juice per meal/snack, adding up to 64 ounces or 8 cups of juice. But don't force-feed yourself like a goose getting prepped for foie gras. If you can only drink 5 ounces this meal, then 5 ounces is all you need.

○ The general rule of thumb is to aim to drink every two hours.

○ Block out a 72-hour time period when you can kick back and relax. For most mortals, that'll be Friday morning through Sunday night. This way, you can make like a hermit and get down to the business of cleansing without an audience.

○ Don't become a couch potato (it's not a safe juicing ingredient). Skip high-intensity workouts, but get your heart pumping daily with some gentle yoga poses or a brisk walk.

○ Finish the last juice two hours before you sleep.

○ Start your cleanse 36 hours before your morning wake-up call. So if your alarm is set for 8 a.m., stop eating at 8 p.m. the night before. If you have a gotta-chew-something-now freak-out, stick with a juicing ingredient such as an apple or a carrot.

○ Try to drink your juice the same time every day to keep cortisol levels low (the stuff that spikes when you're stressed).

Three-Day Cleanse Timetable

Wake-Up Time	8 ounces any drink from the Liquid Diet list (page 103)
Breakfast of Champions (30 minutes later)	8 ounces high-protein drink
Snack (2 hours later)	8 ounces of protein-pumped juice that will also satisfy your sweet tooth
Liquid Lunch (2 hours later)	8 ounces of fiber-filled juice
Afternoon Sugar Craving (2 hours later)	8 ounces of a sweet, high-protein juice
Happy Hour (2 hours later)	8-ounce fruity juice
Not-the-Dog's Dinner (2 hours later)	8 ounces of a hearty, mostly green juice
Sweet Course (2 hours later)	8 ounces of sweetened superfood-based juice
Late-Night Munchies (2 hours later)	8-ounce glass of sleepy-time juice
To Get You through the Night	8 ounces any drink from the Liquid Diet list (page 103)

BACK TO REAL LIFE

Spend at least half the number of days you cleansed to transition back to a more varied diet. Work from the "Meal Plans: What to Eat Before and After Cleansing" (page 99) for each meal and snack. But whatever you eat, think fist-sized portions. After your cleanse, you may realize you don't actually need as much food as you thought you would to get full.

To keep the weight you lost from creeping back, stick with the following eating plan:

EAT FIVE TIMES A DAY: A study in the *American Journal of Epidemiology* established that three healthy meals and two snacks a day cut your risk of gaining weight by 50 percent compared with the three-a-day eaters.

GET YOUR HIGH FIVE (GRAMS OF FIBER PER MEAL): Fiber not only slows digestion, which keeps you feeling full longer and reduces sugar cravings, it also binds to other foods, bulldozing calories out of the body. A USDA study determined that people who consume 24 grams of fiber daily earn a 90-calorie free pass.

DRINK ONE MEAL: One way to keep that "lite" feeling post-cleanse is to bait and switch one meal a day with a cold press juice. The New York Obesity Center at St. Luke's Hospital found that people who replace one meal a day with a healthy liquid drink lose 7 to 8 percent of their body weight in a year, compared with just 3 percent for those who try to eat less food.

LOAD UP ON VEGGIES: Israeli researchers determined that a veggie-heavy meal plan is the most important factor predicting weight loss because these meals give the biggest bang for your caloric buck. Take that, diet soda!

STAY WHOLE: A University of Sydney study found that carb-intense, starchy foods like potatoes and grains have a heavier impact on weight than fats. The healthiest options are the highest-fiber, least-processed versions of these foods (whole wheat breads, pastas and cereals; brown rice instead of white; and whole potatoes with the skin).

RISE AND DINE: Mom was right—breakfast really is the most important meal of the day. It fires up metabolism, making your body less likely to store fat. It's so crucial that University of Massachusetts researchers discovered those who skip the breakfast bar are 4.5 times more likely to be obese.

CLEANSE 3: THE SEVEN-DAY CLEANSE THAT WON'T LEAVE YOU STARVING (NO WIMPS NEED APPLY)

This cleanse separates the dabblers from the serious-minded. It takes dedication, devotion and three-star general organizational skills to stay on a green liquid track for seven days. You'll need to think every meal ahead and be ready for all contingencies (like finding a bathroom in two minutes flat or being able to quip your way out of windy public embarrassment).

Yes, it's hardcore and it's hard, but it's the absolute holy trinity of cleansing: After a week of living on cold press juices, you'll be able to truly reevaluate what, when and why you eat; you'll have effectively liquidated your cravings for salty-sugary-starchy-fatty foods and you'll have lost a hefty amount of weight as well (you'll also look so forward to the opportunity of accidentally swallowing something solid like toothpaste that your teeth will be whiter from all the extra brushing).

Here's what those extra four days of cleansing give you: that rare chance to hit the pause button on the daily insanity that masquerades as your life and connect with yourself. Seven days of cold press juicing means you're not just adding new eating habits, you're really beginning to understand the five Ws of your own personal eating patterns—who you are as an eater, what kinds of foods you munch in different situations, when you're most likely to reach for food, where your eating mostly takes place (car, bad; dining table, good) and why you crave what you crave. This self-assessment is the first step to behavioral change and figuring out an eating plan that truly satisfies you mentally, physically and spiritually.

Taking an extended break from coffee, saturated meats, processed foods, starchy carbs, dairy, refined sugars and, essentially, chewing, can be just the meal ticket to slowing down, checking in with your mind and body and figuring out how to be more in control of something that pretty much dominates your day. The bottom line is hardly anyone eats three to five 100 percent wholesome meals a day or even, for that matter, only when their body signals that it needs fueling. Most of the non-starving population of the world—i.e., probably anyone reading this book—eat when they're feeling happy / sad / bored / tired / angry / stressed / anxious / (insert your emotional eating trigger), because they're feasting on something so delicious that it must be eaten to the bitter end even though their belly is about to burst, simply because it is 1 p.m., and therefore lunchtime (or whatever the time and its corresponding meal is), when they're out with friends, when someone offers them food, when they watch a program on food, when it's a celebration or pretty much anything else...somewhere near the bottom of the list is that they eat simply because they are hungry.

However, let's not sugarcoat the seven-day cleanse—you'll feel hungry. But those hunger pangs are actually mostly mental. Cravings are rarely about nutrients that your body is lacking, even on a cleanse. Yes, you're cutting your daily—possibly, your hourly—caloric intake and you're switching out solids for liquids. As any physics wonk will tell you, solids have more density than liquids. But even though you're drinking your meals, you'll be "eating" a filling amount of calories from ingredients more likely to satisfy, including a healthy dose of protein, fats and fiber. A number of studies concur that eating density-high, low-fat, water-rich, fiber-filled foods like fruits and vegetables are more filling in the long-term than a calorie-limited meat-and-two-veg meal.

The reality is that cravings are usually triggered by the brain. But here's the rub: According to the latest research, giving in to those urges may actually change your brain—especially if your food itch tends to be for processed/fast/junk foods, which have been scientifically designed to offer up a perfect balance of the foods you crave the most: sugar, fat and salt. Foods containing this trio of ingredients seem to stimulate a hot spot in your brain that magnifies the gratification you get from each bite, making you get even more hyped for them. This bliss point moment amps up your brain's response, leading to immediate I-need-another fix and an ugly addictive cycle begins. Case in point: An apple has roughly the same amount of sugar (17 grams) as one of those giant chocolate chip cookies, but while you can easily inhale a stack of cookies, you'll rarely stuff your face with a stack of apples.

What the seven-day cleanse does is put your brain on cold turkey. You'll still be dishing up all of the nutrients your body needs and you'll be feeding your brain healthy versions of sugar, fat and salt, but you'll be taking control of that fat-sugar-salt monkey on your back and satisfying it without feeling deprived ("Junk food, what is it? How does it work? Give me carrots. Yeah, I could really chew my way through a bowl of sweet, crunchy carrots right now.") In short, a seven-day cleanse can turn into a lifetime of happy meals.

The first time really is the hardest. There is such a thing as body memory, so keep in mind for the next time you go on the Seven-Day Cleanse That Won't Leave You Starving, in a minimum of three months, you'll be physically and mentally primed to succeed.

Athletes know that they can improve their game with some conditioning; the same goes for cleansing. You'll need to block out at least three-and-a-half days before (and after) any one week cleanse, which adds up to two weeks of your calendar devoted to a one-week cleanse (yet another reason this kind of cleanse works best when limited to four times a year).

Get diet-prepped by selecting your dishes from each meal in "Meal Plans: What to Eat Before and After Cleansing" (page 99). There are enough choices to keep you going for the full lead-in, but you can stick with the same breakfast, lunch and dinner if your taste buds lean that way.

TIP Log your pre-cleanse onto your calendar to remind you that it is time to start a clean eating plan (see Chapter Four).

SEVEN-DAY CLEANSE SAMPLE MENU

Select a suggested recipe for each meal of the day—sample all seven over the next seven days:

BREAKFAST OF CHAMPIONS

- Aloha (page 134)
- Beat It (page 133)
- Day Breaker (page 132)
- Drink Your Oats (page 136)
- Morning Bracer (page 132)
- Rise and Shine (page 135)
- Un-Coffee Frappe (page 135)

SNACK

- Belly Buster (page 144)
- Energy Boost (page 146)
- Fruitier-Tutti (page 144)
- The Green Hulk (page 139)
- Green Meanies (page 139)
- Mapleberry (page 145)
- Open Sesame (page 141)

LIQUID LUNCH

- 5x5 (page 154)
- The Grass Is Greener (page 153)
- Hippy-Dippy Lunch (page 156)
- Kick in the (Gr)ass (page 152)
- Lunch Combo (page 154)
- Manna (page 157)
- Superfoodie (page 153)

AFTERNOON SUGAR CRAVING

- Afternoon Treat (page 147)
- Coco-Nutty (page 149)
- Cookies and Cream (page 149)
- PM Pick-Me-Up (page 142)
- Sweet Sampler (page 142)
- Snack Attack (page 147)
- Sweeter Than Candy (page 148)

HAPPY HOUR

- Bloody Mary (page 163)
- Citrus Squeeze (page 157)
- Dirty Martini (page 163)
- Liquid Viagra (page 165)
- Mojito (page 162)
- Mudslide (page 164)
- Piña Uncolada (page 164)

NOT-THE-DOG'S DINNER

- Big Gulp (page 170)
- Daily Beast (page 168)
- Happy Healthy Herby (page 170)
- Kitchen Sink (page 169)
- Potluck (page 169)
- Salad Bar (page 168)
- Veggie Delight (page 171)

SWEET COURSE

- Candy Apple (page 177)
- Carrot Cake (page 172)
- Cutie Pie (page 171)
- "Key" Lime Pie (page 178)
- Snickerdoodle (page 178)
- Sourhead (page 175)
- Zucchini Cake (page 175)

- 40 Winks (page 180)
- Cucumber Spa (page 181)
- Fruitopia (page 182)
- Late-Night Refresher (page 182)

- Peppermint Tea (page 180)
- Warm Milk (page 184)
- Warming Zen (page 183)

PRACTICALS

○ Stick with the sample menu. The suggested daily recipes have a balance of go-to ingredients like probiotics, fiber, omega-3s and protein to keep you as rosy-cheeked and energetic as an Olympic skier.

○ Although it's probably simpler to drink the same thing from each category for each meal in terms of preparation and planning of 49 drinks, it's also incredibly boring—which means it'll be tougher to stick to the cleanse for the full 168 hours. The only consistencies in your meals over the next week are trying to stick to a regular time for each drink and making sure that if you decide to go rogue and concoct your own recipe, that you stick with the 80:20 percent vegetable to fruit ratio.

○ Invest in an easy-to-carry cooler and thermos (see "Pimp Your Juicer" on page 40). When it's 5 p.m. and you have to work late, you'll be glad you did.

○ Keep moving. The BMI (Best Moving Index) is to halve your usual routine—if you usually lift 50 pound weights for 20 minutes, switch down to 25 pounders for 10 minutes. If you run for two miles, fast-walk for one. However, if your usual routine involved lying on a couch and watching other people move, go for a 20-minute walk daily.

○ You should be drinking 8 ounces of fresh cold press juice per meal and snack. That amounts to a drink every two hours or so, ideally finishing your final drink around two hours before you go to sleep (see next point).

○ Finish your greens. You may find 8 ounces of drink is too much to finish in one gulp. It's okay to sip and dip throughout the day, but be sure to down all seven juices because you need the full content of calories and nutrients to make it through a full week.

○ Drink from the Liquid Diet (page 103) as needed—you might not need it at all.

○ Plan on making the porcelain bowl your best bud. Go even when you don't feel like you have to. It'll help the swishy juice belly that kicks in around Day Three.

○ Start your cleansing engine 84 hours before the real cleanse begins to ease into the process. See "Meal Plans: What to Eat Before and After Cleansing" on page 99.

○ If you trip up before Day Seven (spoiler alert: this usually happens around Day Three, aka Hump Day), don't beat yourself silly with a limp kale leaf. Simply pick up from where you stumbled.

○ If you broke your cleanse by eating something that you'd be cold pressing into juice anyway, you can count it as one of your fiber drinks such as a snack or your late-night munchies drink.

FRIENDING NON-CLEANSERS

When you're cleansing, seven days is a long time to hang with non-juicing friends. You might decide that it's easier to Howard Hughes the next week and hole up at home. So be it, if your life has that kind of flexibility. But be prepared—seven days is also a long time to be alone with just you and your juicer.

If you're locked into a family and friends plan, it helps if you hook up with a cleansing buddy. There are plenty of people who form juicing circles. Get a group of friends together to juice or even find fellow juicers on social media sites. The point is to have a cheerleading team ready when you are forced to swim with the fast-food eaters.

TIP One way to get rid of the naysayers is to talk about nothing else but your cleanse to anyone who will listen. Possible topics include: This cleanse is amazing; You would not believe how many times I've hit the toilet today; Sorry, I'm feeling a little windy today—can I get a ride with you?

Seven-Day Cleanse Timetable

Wake-Up Time	8 ounces any drink from the Liquid Diet list (page 103)
Breakfast of Champions (30 minutes later)	8 ounces high-protein drink
Snack (2 hours later)	8 ounces of fiber-filled juice that will also curb your morning candy cravings
Liquid Lunch (2 hours later)	8 ounces of superfoods juice
Afternoon Sugar Craving (2 hours later)	8 ounces of a fiber-rich, sweetly satisfying juice
Happy Hour (2 hours later)	8-ounce fruity juice
Not-the-Dog's Dinner (2 hours later)	8 ounces of a filling meal with a healthy fats theme
Sweet Course (2 hours later)	8-ounce treat
Late-Night Munchies (2 hours later)	8-ounce glass of sleepy-time juice that tucks in the fiber
To Get You through the Night	8 ounces any drink from the Liquid Diet list (page 103)

BACK TO REAL LIFE

Head back to the "Meal Plan: What to Eat Before and After Cleansing" (page 99) to ease your body into a more solid menu. As you choose your ingredients, think about the changes you need to make, starting now, to stay in control of your daily diet.

Don't have a meltdown when you regain some of the weight you lost. It's inevitable as you eat more calories. To minimize the pounds, stick with the 4:1 vegetable to fruit ratio and follow these three rules of eating:

1. Eat when you start to get hungry and stop before you feel full.

2. Plan most of your meals in advance to make the healthiest choices possible.

3. Do your best to cut down on the amount of processed foods, artificial sweeteners, alcohol and caffeine in your diet.

SECTION II
Cold Press Juice Recipes

Not all juices have to taste like salad in a glass. What follows is a full roster of fruity, milky, colorful and, of course, green, flavorful cold press juice recipes*. There are enough to easily get you through a one-, three- or seven-day cleanse or a one-a-day-drink for three months without repeating yourself. No matter which juice you brew, you'll get good-for-you benefits in every taste. Not all of the recipes follow the 4:1 ratio because, let's be honest, sometimes, you just want something healthy to satisfy your sweet tooth; however, they all include information on how they can be instantly transformed Superman-style to a superpowered green drink as well as other variations—so no excuses. Drooling permitted.

*Depending on the water content of ingredients, each recipe makes around 8 ounces of juice with no "liquid" ingredients and 16 ounces when fluids are added.

JUICE RULES!

These basic guidelines will keep your from stewing in your own juices:

1. Produce is like fruit: each one is individual. So water content may vary, resulting in a thicker or thinner drink. To adjust, go ahead and drip some more liquid in or squeeze a few more pieces of produce (preferably, vegetables, and most preferably, green vegetables) to get the consistency you want to sip.

2. Remember the Rule of Three. It can be very easy to get carried away and want to add, add, add, especially when there's such a cornucopia of superfoods, powders, herbs, fruits, veggies and leafy greens out there. Unless you know without peeking whether an ingredient needs to be peeled, pitted or pitched as unjuicable, stick with three ingredients when winging a recipe. The results will taste better.

3. If you're not on a strict raw diet, these veggies need a little heat (translation: a two-minute blanch) to put all their nutritional cards on the table (see "Raw or Cooked?" on page 49): asparagus, carrots, kale, peppers, spinach, tomatoes and zucchini. Downside: They'll be slightly mushier for cold pressing and cleanup will be even messier.

4. You don't have to drink the Kool-Aid right away. Newbies might find the 4:1 ratio hard to swallow at first. Rather than pouring the juice down the sink, go ahead and add half a cup of low-sugar fruit like blackberries or raspberries, gradually reducing the fruit as your palate gets used to the green pungency.

5. Be prude(nt) about your ingredients. Nut butters are always 100 percent nutty, nothing added (and yes, that includes salt), vanilla extract is always pure and root vegetables are not into the topless look, so include their greens in the recipe if possible. While any kale will do in any green recipe, if a specific kind is specified, it'll taste all that more lip-smacking.

6. Any juice can instantly be turned into a cooler by pouring it over a cup of ice.

7. So you don't need to play "one of these things is not like the others," all of the recipe ingredients have been grouped in the following order to make pressing decisions easier:

○ Leafy vegetables

○ Herbs

○ Root vegetables

○ Additional vegetables (celery, cucumber, broccoli, tomatoes, etc.)

○ Fruit

○ Seeds and nuts

○ Additional ingredients (proteins, powders, flavorings, sweeteners, etc.)

○ Liquids

8. Don't skip the prep step. Whichever recipe you use, getting your ingredients ready for their close-up juicing is crucial for avoiding emotional (you) and mechanical (your machine) breakdowns. The rules of thumb are to cut down all ingredients to a measurement that easily feeds into the juicer chute (think grape-size). Citrus, kiwi, mangos, pineapples, pomegranates and squash need peeling. Destone/pit/core all fruit; seed and remove rinds from melons; top root vegetables and reserve greens to add separately; bunch and/or roll leafy greens, sprouts, wheatgrass and herbs; and soak nuts in

water at least 12 hours before juicing (keeping water to juice with the nuts); and grind seeds, grains and legumes ("Knife Skills 101" on page 68 has more specific details on prep).

9. All recipes require you to follow the rule of order to avoid clogs—start with the leafy vegetables and then switch back and forth between the hard (root and cruciferous vegetables, seeds/nuts/legumes, apples, citrus, pineapple, etc.) and the soft (fruit, leafy greens, herbs, etc.) produce, finishing with a hard vegetable (see "Get Unclogged" on page 72 for more on how to feed your juicer).

A NOTE ABOUT THE RECIPES

The recipes are divided into seven "mealtimes" (as well as mono juices), but you can skip around depending on your tastebuds, nutritional needs, or whatever you have in your kitchen that day. There are four categories of juices which will be identified with the following symbols:

 GREEN VEGGIE JUICES: These green combos could be called "Beautiful People" drinks because they're the kind of concoctions you see yoga teachers, supermodels and movie stars chugging. Loaded with dark, leafy greens that give cold press juices their big nutritional boost, they make a healthy switch for and/or addition to your daily menu.

 ROOT VEGETABLE JUICES: Juicing these colorful veggies will ensure you get the full rainbow of health benefits with every sip. However, because they tend to have more sweet, starchy ingredients like carrots and beets, which fall high on the GI scale, these juices are not good nutritional substitutes for every meal.

 FRUIT JUICES: While still light on the fruit, these drinks have just enough sweetness to take the green edge off. However, because fruit is their main ingredient, they aren't officially 4:1 ratio recipes (unless you follow the green variation) and are high in fructose—which means sip sparingly as an occasional treat as opposed to a regular meal.

MILKY JUICES: Milky juice sounds like a contradiction in a 100 percent juice fast, but the only thing that milk from nuts, coconuts, seeds, grains and rice have in common with cow's milk is that they're all fluids. Unlike cow's milk, these liquids are heart-friendly, low-calorie and a quick healthy way to get a decadent and delicious dollop of filling protein on your cleanse.

CHAPTER SIX
MONO JUICES

These drinks are specifically designed for the Hardcore Juicer whose palate has adjusted to green, green, and more green and who doesn't need that dollop of fruity sweetness to easily gulp down 8 ounces of healthy sludge on a regular basis. However, their green intensity means that monos are also a good occasional drink for those new to cleansing to make the transition to the world of 4:1 ingredient ratio juicing.

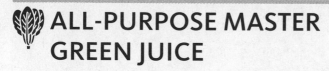
ALL-PURPOSE MASTER GREEN JUICE

2 cups dark, leafy greens (any combination of kale, spinach, Romaine lettuce, watercress, Swiss chard, arugula, mustard greens)

⅓ cup chopped herbs (basil, cilantro, parsley)

1 sprig mint, rosemary, tarragon, oregano, thyme (optional)

2 cups vegetables (cucumber, broccoli, Brussels sprouts, celery)

1 tomato (optional)

One flavoring (1-inch nub fresh ginger, ½ peeled lemon, ½ peeled lime, 1 teaspoon ground cinnamon, 1 teaspoon tumeric, 1 tablespoon nut butter)

Try it this way

Less green: Add 1 cup root vegetables (carrots, beets, parsnips, celeriac root, sweet potato, yam).

More green: Add ½ cup dark, leafy greens.

Sweeter: Add 1 tablespoon of honey, maple syrup, brown rice syrup, Medjool date syrup or stevia leaf powder or extract.

IN THE GREEN

3 leaves dinosaur kale

1 cup chopped Romaine lettuce

½ cup microgreens or any dark green lettuce

½ cup parsley

½ cup basil

2 celery stalks, roughly chopped

1 cucumber

1 teaspoon ground turmeric

¼ teaspoon cayenne pepper

Try it this way

More hardcore: Add 1 cup wheatgrass.

Newbie-friendly: Add 3 carrots and 1 tomato.

A superfood drink: Add 1 teaspoon maca powder.

 # GREEN GODDESS

1 cup watercress

1 cup escarole

1-inch nub fresh ginger

1 broccoli stalk

2 celery stalks

½ cup green beans

1 cucumber

1 lime

Try it this way

More hardcore: Add ½ tablespoon of chlorella powder and ½ cup of bok choy.

Newbie-friendly: Add 1 green apple and 1 teaspoon of blackstrap molasses.

A superfood drink: Add ½ cup of fresh peppermint.

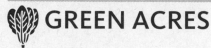 # GREEN ACRES

1 cup spinach

1 cup Swiss chard

½ cup basil

1 zucchini

1 fennel bulb

1 broccoli stalk

1 lemon

Try it this way

More hardcore: Add 1 cup of escarole.

Newbie-friendly: Add 2 kiwis.

A superfood drink: Add 1 tablespoon of chia seeds.

 # GREEN-EYED MONSTER

2 cups spinach

4 kale leaves

½ cup parsley

1 cucumber

1 jalapeño pepper, seeds removed (leave some in if your mouth can take it!)

1 lemon

1 lime

Try it this way

More hardcore: Add ½ cup of Brussels sprouts and ½ head of cabbage.

Newbie-friendly: Add 1 green pear.

A superfood drink: Add 2 teaspoons of honey.

CHAPTER SEVEN
BREAKFAST OF CHAMPIONS

More eye-opening than a cup of Joe, these drinks will get you bright-eyed, bushy-tailed, and ready to face the day. Green juice is a healthy way to wake up your body. Liquids are easier on your digestive system in the morning than solid foods are and fill you up without the residual stuffed, sluggish feeling that can come with a more standard breakfast fare. Good morning, sunshine!

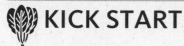 KICK START

6 curly kale leaves	1 tomato
½ cup arugula	1 green pepper
¼ cup herbs (cilantro, parsley, chives, basil, sorrel, mint and/ or lemon balm)	1 lemon
	1 tablespoon protein powder
1-inch nub fresh ginger	½ teaspoon Medjool date syrup

Try it this way

Rooty: Add 2 beets and a small kohlrabi.

Milky: Switch the protein powder for ½ cup to 1 cup of almond milk.

Fruity: Add 2 tart apples.

"GREEN TEA"

1 cup wheatgrass	½ head cabbage
4 kale leaves	½ cup broccoli

Try it this way

Rooty: Add 1 parsnip.

Milky: Add 1 cup of sprouted grain milk.

Fruity: Add ½ honeydew melon.

MORNING BRACER

4 medium carrots

1 small golden beet

1 orange

1 tomato

1 tablespoon nut butter

1 tablespoon coconut oil

½ tablespoon ground turmeric

Try it this way

Milky: Substitute 1 cup of coconut water for the coconut oil.

Green: Add 5 collard green leaves and 1 cup of tatsoi.

Fruity: Add 1 red apple.

DAY BREAKER

1 sweet potato

2 large carrots

½ sweet onion

2 celery stalks

½ cucumber

1 tablespoon hemp seeds

Splash of any vinegar

Try it this way

Milky: Substitute 1 cup of nut milk for the hemp seeds.

Green: Add 2 cups of spinach.

Fruity: Add 1 green apple and 1 red apple.

BEAT IT

3 red beets

1-inch nub fresh ginger

½ cucumber

1 tablespoon sunflower butter

Splash of any fruit vinegar

Try it this way

Milky: Add ½ cup of brown rice milk.

Green: Add 2 cups of Swiss chard.

Fruity: Add 1 cup of pineapple.

SUNRISE SURPRISE

½ cup spinach

¼ cup mint leaves

1 cup strawberries

½ cup pineapple

1 tablespoon hemp powder

1 tablespoon sunflower seeds

Try it this way

Milky: Substitute ½ cup of coconut water for ¼ cup of the pineapple.

Green: Add ½ cup of sugar peas in their pods and 1 cup of bok choy.

Rooty: Substitute 3 carrots and 1-inch nub of fresh ginger for the pineapple.

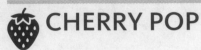

CHERRY POP

¼ cup radicchio	2 apples
1 beet	1 cup cherries
2 tomatoes	1 lime
1 cucumber	

Try it this way

Milky: Substitute 1 cup of walnut milk for the apples.

Green: Add 1 cup spinach, ½ cup tatsoi and 5 broccoli stalks.

Rooty: Add 2 carrots.

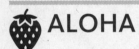

ALOHA

1 cup spinach	1 tablespoon chia seeds
1 cup tatsoi	1 tablespoon cocoa powder
1 cup pineapple	1 teaspoon Five Spice powder
½ cup mango	

Try it this way

Milky: Add ½ cup of coconut water.

Green: Add ½ cup of wheatgrass.

Rooty: Add 2 carrots.

RISE AND SHINE

1 orange

1 apple

1 slice pineapple

1 apricot

½ lemon

1-inch turmeric root

1 tablespoon bee pollen

Try it this way

Milky: Substitute 1 cup of sprouted grain milk for the pineapple.

Green: Add 2 cups of spinach.

Rooty: Substitute 9 carrots for the apple.

 # UN-COFFEE FRAPPE

½ cup blueberries

1 tablespoon hazel or macadamia nuts

1 tablespoon whey protein powder

1 teaspoon ground cinnamon

¼ teaspoon ground nutmeg

1 tablespoon stevia (optional)

1 cup hemp milk

Try it this way

Green: Add 1 cup of chicory greens and 1 cup of spinach.

Fruity: Add ¼ cup of peaches.

Rooty: Add 2 beets.

STRAWBERRY MILKSHAKE

½ cup strawberries

½ tablespoon agave nectar

½ teaspoon ground cinnamon

½ teaspoon vanilla extract

1 cup almond milk

Try it this way

Green: Add 1 cup of spinach and 6 curly kale leaves.

Fruity: Add 1 orange.

Rooty: Add 2 carrots.

DRINK YOUR OATS

2 apples

2 teaspoons maple syrup

1 cup sprouted oat milk

Try it this way

Green: Add 2 cups of spinach.

Fruity: Substitute ½ cup of berries (your choice) for 1 apple.

Rooty: Add a 1-inch nub of ginger.

CHAPTER EIGHT
SNACKS

It's unhealthy snacking, rather than the munchies themselves, that leads to weight gain and mood swings. The National Weight Control Registry has determined if you go more than four hours without eating, you end up on a fattening cycle where your blood sugar levels drop, leaving you starving, not just a little cranky and tired, and more likely to pig out on your next meal. These sugar-quenchers are designed to keep you snacking happy by giving you the most bang per sip, keeping you healthily energized and feeling partly full until your next meal.

PEANUT BUTTER CUP

2 cups spinach

1 tablespoon chia seeds

¼ cup chocolate protein powder

1 tablespoon peanut butter

1 tablespoon honey

Try it this way

Rooty: Add 1 small sweet potato.

Milky: Add 1 cup vanilla-infused almond milk.

Fruity: Add 5 fresh cherries.

 # SWEET GREENS

2 cups spinach

1 cup green beans

½ cup red bell pepper

1 tablespoon cacao powder

1 teaspoon stevia

½ teaspoon ground cinnamon

Splash of apple cider vinegar

Try it this way

Rooty: Substitute 1 rutabaga for the pepper.

Milky: Add 1 cup chocolate-infused almond milk.

Fruity: Add 1 pear.

THE GREEN HULK

3 dinosaur kale leaves

3 curly kale leaves

½ cup escarole

½ cup Swiss chard

4 asparagus stalks

1 teaspoon ground flaxseed

⅛ teaspoon ground cumin

Try it this way

Rooty: Add 1 radish and 1 tomato.

Milky: Add 1 cup of rice milk.

Fruity: Add 2 oranges.

GREEN MEANIES

1 cup spinach

1 cup Swiss chard

5 kale leaves

½ cup parsley

¼ cup herbs (cilantro, chives, basil, sorrel, mint and/or lemon balm)

1 teaspoon fresh thyme

2 broccoli stalks

2 asparagus stalks

1 cucumber

1 lime

Try it this way

Rooty: Add 4 jicama bulbs.

Milky: Add ½ cup of sprouted grain milk.

Fruity: Add 1 apple and 1 pear.

GINGERBREAD

2-inch nub fresh ginger

2 carrots

½ cucumber

1 tablespoon vanilla protein powder

¼ teaspoon ground cinnamon

Try it this way

Milky: Substitute 1 cup of almond milk for the ½ cucumber.

Green: Add 2 cups of spinach.

Fruity: Add 1 grapefruit.

WHAT'S UP DOC?

9 carrots

½-inch nub fresh ginger

1 orange

1 pineapple slice

½ lemon

1 tablespoon ground turmeric

$\frac{1}{16}$ teaspoon cayenne pepper

Try it this way

Milky: Add ½ cup of almond milk.

Green: Add 2 cups of collard leaves.

Fruity: Add 2 apricots.

TRAIL MIX

3 carrots

2 beets

½ butternut squash

½ cup cranberries

¼ cup almond butter

1 tablespoon cacao nibs

1 tablespoon wheat germ

1 tablespoon maple syrup

½ teaspoon ground cinnamon

Try it this way

Milky: Add 1 cup of sprouted oat milk.

Green: Add 2 cups of Romaine lettuce.

Fruity: Add ½ cup of blueberries.

OPEN SESAME

2 beets

2 carrots

5 cauliflower florets

1 tablespoon sesame butter/ seeds or tahini

1 teaspoon miso paste

1 cup water

Try it this way

Milky: Substitute 1 cup of sesame seed milk for the water.

Green: Add ½ cup of green beans.

Fruity: Add 1 apple.

PM PICK-ME-UP

1 golden beet

1 radish

3 carrots

½-inch nub fresh ginger

4 celery stalks

1 tomato

½ cucumber

1 medium pear

½ cup sprouts

1 tablespoon sunflower butter

Splash of apple cider vinegar

Try it this way

Milky: Substitute nut milk for the sunflower butter.

Green: Add 5 kale leaves and ½ cup of green beans.

Fruity: Substitute 1 plum for the cucumber.

SWEET SAMPLER

3 parsnips

3 carrots

1 celery stalk

½ cup green beans

1 apple

Try it this way

Milky: Add 1 cup of sprouted grain milk.

Green: Substitute ½ head of green cabbage for the green beans.

Fruity: Add 5 strawberries and 2 rhubarb stalks.

CHOCOLATE SILK

3 leaves kale

1 beet

2 carrots

1 teaspoon hemp seeds

1 teaspoon ground flaxseed

1 heaping tablespoon chocolate protein powder

1 tablespoon cacao nibs

1 teaspoon ground cinnamon

2 teaspoons stevia (chocolate, if possible)

Try it this way

Milky: Add 1 cup of almond milk.

Green: Add 2 cups of Romaine lettuce.

Fruity: Add 1 orange.

SWEET POTATO PIE

1 medium sweet potato

3 medium carrots

1-inch nub fresh ginger

2 celery stalks

1 red pepper

1 tablespoon pumpkin seeds

1 tablespoon whey protein powder

½ teaspoon ground nutmeg

1 teaspoon ground cinnamon

Splash of any vinegar

Try it this way

Milky: Substitute 1 cup of coconut water for the red pepper.

Green: Add 2 cups of spinach.

Fruity: Add 1 orange.

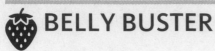

BELLY BUSTER

¼ cup parsley

2 pears

3 pink grapefruits

1 tablespoon ground flaxseed

Try it this way

Milky: Substitute 1 cup of coconut water for 2 grapefruits.

Green: Substitute 1 cup of Swiss chard and 1 cup of spinach for the pears.

Rooty: Add 1 sweet potato.

FRUITIER-TUTTI

1 cucumber

¼ head cauliflower

¼ cup parsley

¼ cup basil

1 apple

1 pomegranate

2 plums (red or black)

½ cup black cherries

½ cup strawberries

1 tablespoon lime juice

Try it this way

Milky: Add ½ cup of brown rice milk.

Green: Add 1 cup of spinach and substitute 1 cup of broccoli and 1 tomato for the cherries.

Rooty: Substitute 2 beets and 1 tomato for the black cherries.

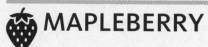

MAPLEBERRY

¼ head red cabbage

1 cucumber

2 apples

1 cup blueberries

1 tablespoon maple syrup

¼ lemon

Try it this way

Milky: Substitute 1 cup of sprouted grain milk for the cucumber.

Green: Add 1 cup of spinach and 1 cup of Swiss chard.

Rooty: Substitute 1 beet and 1 tomato for 1 apple.

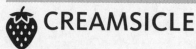

CREAMSICLE

4 carrots

3 celery stalks

1 Golden Delicious apple

2 oranges

1 apricot

Try it this way

Milky: Substitute ½ cup of brown rice milk for the apple.

Green: Add 1 cup of broccoli and 1 cup of spinach.

Rooty: Add 1 sweet potato.

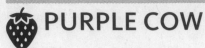

PURPLE COW

¼ head red cabbage

¼ cup radicchio

1 apple

1 cup blueberries

½ lemon

1 tablespoon cocoa powder

1 teaspoon ground cinnamon

Try it this way

Milky: Substitute 1 cup of almond milk for 1 apple.

Green: Add 1 cup of Romaine lettuce and 6 kale leaves.

Rooty: Add 2 carrots.

ENERGY BOOST

½ watermelon

5 oranges

1 cup pineapple

1 lime

1 tablespoon wheat germ

Try it this way

Milky: Substitute 1 cup of sprouted grain milk for 3 oranges and the wheat germ.

Green: Add 6 kale leaves and 1 cup of wheatgrass.

Rooty: Substitute 2 beets and 1 tomato for 3 oranges.

AFTERNOON TREAT

1 cup spinach	½ lime
2 kiwis	2 tablespoons ground flaxseed
1 apple	1 teaspoon honey

Try it this way

Milky: Add ½ cup of coconut water.

Green: Add 1 cup of Romaine leaves and substitute 1 cucumber for 1 kiwi.

Rooty: Substitute 2 beets for the kiwi.

 # SNACK ATTACK

3 oranges	1 lime
1 cup grapes	1 teaspoon ground cinnamon

Try it this way

Milky: Substitute ½ cup of almond milk for 2 oranges.

Green: Add 1 cup of mustard greens and 5 leaves of kale, and substitute 4 celery stalks for the grapes.

Rooty: Add 1-inch nub of fresh ginger.

SWEETER THAN CANDY

½ cup Swiss chard

2 apples

½ cantaloupe

½ honeydew melon

1 tablespoon Medjool date syrup

Try it this way

Milky: Add ½ cup of coconut water.

Green: Add 6 kale leaves and 1 cup of spinach.

Rooty: Add 2 carrots and 1 tomato.

 # GOIN' NUTZ

1 tablespoon almond butter

1 tablespoon peanut butter

1 tablespoon honey

pinch of ground cloves

½ cup cashew milk

½ cup pistachio milk

Try it this way

Green: Add ½ cup of parsley, ½ cucumber and ½ head of cabbage.

Fruity: Substitute 2 apples for half of the nut milk.

Rooty: Substitute 4 carrots for half of the nut butter.

COCO-NUTTY

½ cup cauliflower

1 mango

1 apple

1 tablespoon sunflower seed butter

1 cup coconut water

Try it this way

Green: Add 1 cup of spinach, ½ cup of arugula and 5 kale leaves.

Fruity: Substitute 1 cup of pineapple for ½ cup of coconut water.

Rooty: Substitute 1 sweet potato for the cauliflower.

COOKIES AND CREAM

1 head cauliflower

1 tablespoon cashew butter

2 tablespoons carob powder

1 tablespoon honey

1 teaspoon vanilla extract

½ cup brown rice milk

½ cup coconut water

Try it this way

Green: Add 6 curly kale leaves, ½ cup of spinach and ½ head of cabbage.

Fruity: Add 1 cup of raspberries.

Rooty: Add 1 sweet potato.

CHAPTER NINE
LIQUID LUNCH

Drinking your midday meal is a convenient way to add nutrient-dense foods to your diet on a regular basis. Eating a pound of greens in one sitting sounds about as appealing as, well, eating a pound of greens . But jazz it up with spices, nut milks, fruit and other vegetables, and stick a straw in it—and you've got yourself a meal that's more filling than a sandwich, healthier than a salad and the quicker to consume than any fast food, leaving you more time to enjoy your lunch hour.

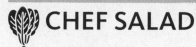

CHEF SALAD

1 cup spinach	1 cucumber
1 cup arugula	½ cup sprouts
1 green bell pepper	1 tablespoon wheat germ
1 tomato	Splash of any fruit vinegar
2 carrots	

Try it this way

Rooty: Add ¼ cup red onion.

Milky: Substitute ½ cup of sprouted grain milk for the wheat germ.

Fruity: Substitute 10 green grapes for the cucumber.

 # BIG THREE

1 cup arugula or dandelion greens	1 tablespoon ground flaxseed
5 kale leaves	1 teaspoon honey
1 tablespoon chia seeds	1 tablespoon protein powder
	1 cup kombucha tea

Try it this way

Rooty: Add 1 small beet.

Milky: Substitute 1 cup of soy milk for the kombucha tea.

Fruity: Add 4 strawberries.

SPICY MEXICAN GREEN

3 collard green leaves

¼ cup cilantro

2 tomatoes

½ medium cucumber

1 lime

1 small jalapeño pepper, seeded

1 tablespoon cacao powder

Try it this way

Rooty: Add 1 carrot.

Milky: Add ½ cup of pumpkin seed milk.

Fruity: Add 1 green apple.

KICK IN THE (GR)ASS

5 curly kale leaves

1 cup dandelion greens or arugula

½ cup wheatgrass

½ cup parsley

¼ cup herbs (cilantro, chives, basil, sorrel, mint and/or lemon balm)

½ cup sprouts

1-inch nub fresh ginger

1 large cucumber

4 celery stalks

4 asparagus stalks

1 lemon

Try it this way

Rooty: Substitute 1 cup of celeriac root for the celery.

Milky: Substitute ½ cup of coconut water for the cucumber.

Fruity: Substitute 1 cup of green grapes for the cucumber.

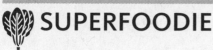

SUPERFOODIE

4 kale leaves	2 broccoli stalks
¼ cup Brussels sprouts	1 tomato
¼ red cabbage head	1 tablespoon carob powder
4 celery stalks	1 tablespoon coconut oil
2 asparagus stalks	Splash of any vinegar

Try it this way

Rooty: Add 2 carrots.

Milky: Add ½ cup of aloe vera juice.

Fruity: Substitute 1 plum for the Brussels sprouts.

THE GRASS IS GREENER

1 head romaine lettuce	¼ cup mint
¼ cup wheat grass	3 cauliflower florets
¼ cup parsley	1 cup kombucha tea

Try it this way

Rooty: Substitute 3 carrots for the cauliflower.

Milky: Substitute ½ cup of soy milk for ½ cup of kombucha tea.

Fruity: Add ½ cup of raspberries.

5X5

5 kale leaves

5 Brussels sprouts

5 cauliflower florets

5 pieces red bell pepper

5 ounces kombucha tea

Try it this way

Rooty: Substitute 1 small beet for the red pepper.

Milky: Add ¼ cup of nut milk.

Fruity: Add 5 green grapes.

 # LUNCH COMBO

1 cup bok choy

1 cup tatsoi

½ cup Thai basil

½ cup sprouts

1-inch nub fresh ginger

3 celery stalks

½ cup green beans

1 tablespoon miso paste

Splash of rice vinegar

Try it this way

Rooty: Add ½ cup red bell pepper and 1 small tomato.

Milky: Substitute 1 cup soy milk for the miso paste.

Fruity: Substitute 2 plums for the celery.

CURRY CHAI

1 cup spinach	1 tablespoon pumpkin seeds
2 golden beets	1 teaspoon curry powder
3 large carrots	1 teaspoon ground cinnamon
1-inch nub fresh ginger	½ teaspoon ground cardamom
1 Golden Delicious apple	½ teaspoon ground allspice
1 orange	½ teaspoon ground cloves
1 tablespoon Medjool date syrup	¼ teaspoon ground nutmeg

Try it this way

Milky: Add 1 cup of coconut water.

Green: Add 5 dinosaur kale leaves and 1 cup of mustard greens or arugula.

Fruity: Add ½ mango and 2 tomatoes.

LEMONADE

2 golden beets	2 Golden Delicious apples
2 yellow carrots	2 lemons
½ cucumber	1 tablespoon honey
2 Asian pears	

Try it this way

Milky: Substitute ½ cup of rice milk for the cucumber.

Green: Add 1 head of green cabbage.

Fruity: Substitute 1 yellow grapefruit for the cucumber.

TWILIGHT

1 cup red Swiss chard	1 apple
3 beets	2 rhubarb stalks
1 parsnip	½ cup strawberries
1 tomato	

Try it this way

Milky: Add 1 cup of brown rice milk.

Green: Add 1 cup of red cabbage.

Fruity: Add 2 oranges.

 # HIPPY-DIPPY LUNCH

2 beets	1 apple
1 radish	1 tablespoon hemp seeds
1 carrot	1 tablespoon sunflower seeds
2 cups sprouts	1 tablespoon honey
2 tomatoes	1 cup kombucha tea

Try it this way

Milky: Substitute 1 cup of sprouted grain for the sprouts and kombucha, and add 1 tablespoon of miso paste.

Green: Add 6 kale leaves and 1 cup of wheatgrass.

Fruity: Substitute ½ cup of blueberries for the radish.

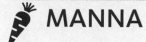 MANNA

4 carrots	½-inch nub fresh ginger
1 beet	1 tablespoon sunflower seeds
½ celeriac root	1 tablespoon hemp seeds
2 small jicama bulbs	1 tablespoon pumpkin seeds
1 apple	1 tablespoon honey

Try it this way

Milky: Add 1 cup of sprouted grain milk.

Green: Add 5 kale leaves and 1 cup of spinach.

Fruity: Add 1 cup of pomegranate seeds.

CITRUS SQUEEZE

2-inch nub fresh ginger	2 grapefruits
3 cups cranberries	1 cup pineapple juice
2 oranges	2 limes

Try it this way

Milky: Substitute 1 cup of brown rice milk for 1 grapefruit and 1 orange.

Green: Add 1 cup of wheatgrass and 1 cup of spinach.

Rooty: Substitute 2 carrots and 2 beets for the cranberries.

HAWAIIAN PUNCH

1 apple

1 apricot

1 guava

1 passion fruit

1 cup pineapple

Try it this way

Milky: Substitute ½ cup coconut water for ½ cup of pineapple.

Green: Add 1 cup of wheatgrass and 1 cup of bok choy.

Rooty: Substitute 1 sweet potato and 1 beet for the apple and apricot.

 # KICK-ASS LEMONADE

3 lemons

½ teaspoon cayenne pepper

2 tablespoons agave syrup or honey

6 ounces aloe vera juice or water

Try it this way

Milky: Substitute coconut water for aloe vera juice.

Green: Add 1 cup of wheat grass and 6 curly kale leaves.

Rooty: Add 2 carrots and a 1-inch nub of fresh ginger.

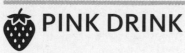 # PINK DRINK

1 beet	1 apple
½ cucumber	1 grapefruit

Try it this way

Milky: Add ½ cup of coconut water.

Green: Add 1 cup of spinach and 1 cup of red Swiss chard.

Rooty: Add ½ of a celeriac root.

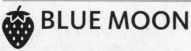 # BLUE MOON

½ cup mint leaves	1 cup blackberries
5 broccoli stalks	1 cup black grapes
1 cup blueberries	1 pear

Try it this way

Milky: Substitute ½ cup of coconut water for ½ cup of blueberries or blackberries.

Green: Add 2 cups of red Swiss chard.

Rooty: Substitute 1 beet for the pear.

CHAPTER TEN
HAPPY HOUR

No liquor doesn't mean no libations. You won't miss the buzz with these mocktails. You lose the booze, but not the flavor. The recipes below are as refreshing as gin and tonics, as complex as a whiskey sour, and as alcoholic as... kale juice. So you can eat, drink and be merry and still be able to drive home.

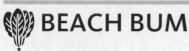 BEACH BUM

1 cup spinach

¼ cup basil

1 cup pineapple

1 lime

1 cup coconut water

Try it this way

Rooty: Add 1 small golden beet.

Milky: Substitute ½ cup of almond milk for ½ cup of coconut water.

Fruity: Add 1 mango and 1 apricot.

GREEN CHARTREUSE

1 cup dandelion leaves or arugula

1 cup spinach

1 fennel bulb

½ cup green beans

1 teaspoon chlorella

½ cup aloe vera juice

Try it this way

Rooty: Add 2 jicama bulbs.

Milky: Substitute ¼ cup of nut milk for ¼ cup of aloe vera juice.

Fruity: Add 1 lime.

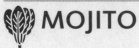 # MOJITO

1 cup arugula	½ cup mint
1 cup spinach	2 limes
2 cucumbers	1 tablespoon honey
¼ cup sugar peas in their pods	

Try it this way

Rooty: Add 1-inch nub of fresh ginger.

Milky: Add 1 cup of coconut water.

Fruity: Substitute 1 cup of watermelon for 1 cucumber.

 # BLUE BLOOD

1 large kale leaf	½ cup blueberries
1 beet	1 cup aloe vera juice
1 purple turnip	

Try it this way

Milky: Substitute 1 cup of coconut water for the aloe vera juice.

Green: Add 1 cup of Swiss chard.

Fruity: Add 10 purple grapes.

BLOODY MARY

¼ cup parsley

3 carrots

1 celeriac root

1-inch nub horseradish root or 1 tablespoon 100 percent horseradish

1 yellow onion

3 tomatoes

½ cucumber

1 lime

1 teaspoon cayenne pepper

Try it this way

Milky: Add ½ cup of brown rice milk.

Green: Add 1 cup of spinach and 1 cup of watercress.

Fruity: Add 1 red apple.

DIRTY MARTINI

1 turnip

1 fennel bulb

1 cucumber

8 celery stalks

1 teaspoon blackstrap molasses

½ cup water

Try it this way

Milky: Substitute ½ cup of nut milk for the water.

Green: Add 6 kale leaves and 1 cup of dandelion leaves or arugula.

Fruity: Add 1 pear.

PIÑA UNCOLADA

½ cup green beans

1 cup pineapple

1 Granny Smith apple

2 teaspoons maple syrup

1 cup coconut water

Try it this way

Green: Add 2 cups of spinach and substitute ½ cucumber and ½ cup of broccoli rabe for the apple.

Fruity: Substitute 1 mango and 1 kiwi for the apple.

Rooty: Add 2 carrots.

MUDSLIDE

½ cup cherries

1 apple

1 tablespoon ground flaxseed

2 tablespoons carob powder

2 tablespoons cacao powder

1 tablespoon Medjool date syrup

1 cup sprouted grain milk

Try it this way

Green: Add 1 head of Romaine lettuce and substitute ½ cup of broccoli for the apple.

Fruity: Add ½ cup of strawberries and 1 tomato.

Rooty: Substitute 2 beets for the apple.

LIQUID VIAGRA

¼ cup mint or basil

2 celery stalks

½ cup watermelon

1 tablespoon maca powder

1 tablespoon honey

1 teaspoon ground cardamom

1 pinch chili powder or hot pepper flakes

1 cup almond milk

Try it this way

Green: Add 2 cups of spinach.

Fruity: Substitute 1 orange for ¼ cup of watermelon.

Rooty: Add 1 sweet potato.

CHAPTER ELEVEN
NOT-THE-DOG'S DINNER

Finding a savory juice (can you juice a steak?) that tastes like something other than salsa and that isn't too sweet for dinner can be tricky. These recipes are as varied in taste as a full-course main meal and are just as filling. The better news is that they can be thrown together more quickly. The best news is that even when you go back to solids, you can use these—or any juice recipe—as a concentrated base for soups and sauces.

KISSING A COW

1 cup wheatgrass	½ cup alfalfa sprouts
½ cup spinach	2 large carrots
1 cup parsley	3 celery stalks
¼ cup herbs (cilantro, chives, basil, sorrel, mint and/or lemon balm)	Splash of apple cider vinegar

Try it this way

Rooty: Substitute 1 beet for 1 carrot.

Milky: Add 1 cup of coconut water.

Fruity: Add 1 peach.

SWEET AND SOUR

1 cup spinach	2 yellow grapefruits
1 cup watercress	1 apricot
¼ cup green beans	1 tablespoon honey
¼ cup sugar peas in their pods	Splash of any vinegar
2 zucchini	

Try it this way

Rooty: Add 1-inch nub of fresh ginger.

Milky: Substitute 1 cup of rice milk for 1 grapefruit.

Fruity: Add ½ cup of strawberries and 2 rhubarb stalks.

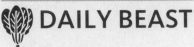 # DAILY BEAST

5 kale leaves	½ cup basil
½ cup spinach	5 grapes
½ cup Brussels sprouts	1 orange

Try it this way

Rooty: Add 1 carrot.

Milky: Add ½ cup of coconut water.

Fruity: Substitute 1 apple for 3 grapes.

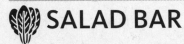 # SALAD BAR

2 kale leaves	¼ cup sugar peas in their pods
¼ head cabbage	¼ head cauliflower
3 sprigs parsley	½ lemon
1 broccoli stalk	

Try it this way

Rooty: Add 1 radish.

Milky: Add 1 cup of sprouted grain milk.

Fruity: Add 1 apple.

KITCHEN SINK

5 kale leaves

1 cup microgreens or dark green lettuce

½ butternut squash

1 carrot

1-inch nub fresh ginger

1 pear

1 red bell pepper

2 tomatoes

3 celery stalks

¼ cup sugar peas in their pods

½ cup sprouts

¼ cup herbs (cilantro, parsley, chives, basil, sorrel, mint and/or lemon balm)

½ lime

1 tablespoon nutritional yeast flakes

Try it this way

Rooty: Add 1 parsnip.

Milky: Add 1 cup of coconut water.

Fruity: Add 1 red apple.

POTLUCK

½ head Romaine lettuce

10 Brussels sprouts

½ cup parsley

¼ cup herbs (cilantro, chives, basil, sorrel, mint and/or lemon balm)

3 sprigs dill

2 beets

½ cucumber

2 celery stalks

1 orange

Try it this way

Rooty: Add 3 carrots.

Milky: Add 1 cup of sunflower seed milk.

Fruity: Add 1 apple.

HAPPY HEALTHY HERBY

½ cup flat-leaf parsley

½ cup cilantro

¼ cup mint

¼ cup lemon balm

1 honeydew melon

1 tablespoon chia seeds

1 tablespoon honey

Splash of any vinegar

Try it this way

Rooty: Add 3 jicama bulbs.

Milky: Add 1 cup of coconut water.

Fruity: Add 1 apricot.

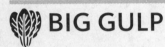 # BIG GULP

3 kale leaves

¼ head cabbage

1-inch nub fresh ginger

½ mango

½ lemon

Pinch of cayenne pepper

Try it this way

Rooty: Add 2 carrots.

Milky: Add 1 cup walnut milk.

Fruity: Add the rest of the mango.

VEGGIE DELIGHT

2 red beets

1 butternut squash

1 carrot

1 tomato

1 red bell pepper

½ cup green beans

1 Golden Delicious apple

Try it this way

Milky: Add 1 cup of rice milk.

Green: Add 1 cup of Swiss chard and 1 cup of spinach.

Fruity: Add 1 orange.

CUTIE PIE

1 butternut squash

2 golden beets

1 parsnip

4 peaches

1 tablespoon pumpkin seeds

1 tablespoon honey

1 teaspoon ground cinnamon

Try it this way

Milky: Add 1 cup of coconut water.

Green: Add 1 head of green cabbage.

Fruity: Add 1 Golden Delicious apple.

MOOD INDIGO

¼ head red cabbage

5 sprigs cilantro

2 carrots

1-inch nub fresh ginger

2 apples

½ lemon

Try it this way

Milky: Add ½ cup of sprouted grain milk.

Green: Add 6 Swiss chard leaves and ¼ cup of tatsoi leaves.

Fruity: Add ½ cup of blueberries.

CARROT CAKE

1 golden beet

5 large carrots

½-inch nub fresh ginger

1 zucchini

1 medium pear

1 tablespoon nut butter

1 teaspoon ground cinnamon

1 tablespoon Medjool date syrup

Try it this way

Milky: Substitute 1 cup of walnut milk for the nut butter.

Green: Add 1 cup of Swiss chard and 1 cup of green cabbage.

Fruity: Add 1 Granny Smith apple.

NEAPOLITAN

1 head red cabbage	3 cups cranberries
2 beets	2 limes
2 parsnips	½ cup water
2 jicama bulbs	

Try it this way

Milky: Substitute ½ cup of rice milk for the water.

Green: Add ½ head of green cabbage.

Fruity: Add 1 Ruby Red grapefruit.

CHAPTER TWELVE
SWEET COURSE

"Clean eating" and "dessert" don't look like they should be in the same sentence. But a University of Minnesota School of Public Health in Minneapolis determined that making certain foods forbidden is practically guaranteed to make you crave those tastes all the more. These mouthwatering drinks will healthfully satisfy your sweet tooth. Life is sweet!

ZUCCHINI CAKE

5 curly kale leaves

1 cup spinach

1-inch nub fresh ginger

½ cucumber

1 zucchini

2 green pears

½ lemon

1 tablespoon carob powder

1 tablespoon Medjool date syrup

¼ teaspoon ground nutmeg

Try it this way

Rooty: Substitute 1 beet for 1 pear.

Milky: Substitute 1 cup of nut milk for the cucumber.

Fruity: Substitute 1 apple for the cucumber.

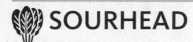 SOURHEAD

4 curly kale leaves

¼ cup mint

2 lemons

1 lime

1 tablespoon chlorophyll powder

1 teaspoon stevia

Try it this way

Rooty: Add 1-inch nub of fresh ginger.

Milky: Add 1 cup of rice milk.

Fruity: Add ½ cup of raspberries.

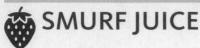

SMURF JUICE

1 cup cilantro	½ cup raspberries
½ cup strawberries	1 mango
½ cup blueberries	1 lime

Try it this way

Milky: Substitute 1 cup of almond milk for the lime.

Green: Add 6 dinosaur kale leaves and substitute ½ cup of green beans for the mango.

Rooty: Substitute 2 carrots for the mango.

TROPICAL DELIGHT

1 head cabbage	1 clementine
1-inch nub fresh ginger	½ cup pineapple
1 mango	1 tablespoon lime
1 kiwi	1 teaspoon ground cardamom
6 strawberries	

Try it this way

Milky: Substitute ¼ cup of coconut water for 3 strawberries.

Green: Add ½ cup of spinach and 1 fennel bulb.

Rooty: Add 2 carrots.

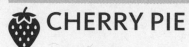

CHERRY PIE

1 cup Swiss chard

2 celery stalks

½ cucumber

1 cup black cherries

½ cup strawberries

1 green apple

1 lime

Try it this way

Milky: Substitute ½ cup of sprouted grain milk for the lime.

Green: Add ½ head of cabbage and ¼ cup of mint leaves.

Rooty: Substitute 3 beets for the strawberries.

CANDY APPLE

½ cup red bell pepper

1 tomato

1 Golden Delicious apple

1 red apple

1 Granny Smith apple

½ cup strawberries

1 teaspoon ground cinnamon

Try it this way

Milky: Substitute ½ cup of coconut water for the strawberries.

Green: Add 2 cups of red Swiss chard.

Rooty: Substitute 2 carrots for the strawberries.

SNICKERDOODLE

½ head cauliflower

½ cucumber

1 apple

2 tablespoons peanut butter

2 tablespoons carob powder

1 teaspoon ground cinnamon

1 cup brown rice milk

Try it this way

Green: Add 1 cup of wheatgrass and 1 cup of bok choy.

Fruity: Substitute 1 orange for the cucumber.

Rooty: Substitute 2 carrots for ½ of the cucumber.

"KEY" LIME PIE

½ head cabbage

1 celery stalk

½ cup honeydew melon

1 apple

3 limes

1 cup coconut water

Try it this way

Green: Add 5 kale leaves and 1 cup of wheatgrass and substitute ½ cup of green beans for the honeydew melon.

Fruity: Substitute 1 mango for 1 lime.

Rooty: Substitute 3 carrots for the celery.

CHAPTER THIRTEEN
LATE-NIGHT MUNCHIES

You've been told eating before bed is a no-no. But research on sleep disorders shows that healthy snacking before bed actually helps your zzzz's. The trick is to munch on fare that won't spike your blood sugar, incite cravings or pack on pounds. Any of these light-but-filling juices should tide you over till morning.

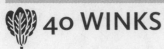 40 WINKS

½ cup spinach

½ head Romaine lettuce

¼ cup sugar peas in their pods

8 celery stalks

2 oranges

1 lemon

Try it this way

Rooty: Substitute 2 beets for the oranges.

Milky: Add 1 cup coconut water.

Fruity: Substitute 2 plums for the parsley.

PEPPERMINT TEA

1 cup spinach

2 celery stalks

¼ cup mint leaves

1 cup watermelon

Try it this way

Rooty: Add ½ cup of celeriac root.

Milky: Substitute ½ cup of sprouted grain milk for ½ cup watermelon.

Fruity: Add 1 kiwi.

CUCUMBER SPA

1 head of Romaine lettuce

1 cup parsley

2 cucumbers

1 lime

3 tablespoons honey

Try it this way

Rooty: Add 1-inch nub of fresh ginger.

Milky: Substitute ½ cup of rice milk for 1 cucumber.

Fruity: Add 1 cup berries.

 # HAPPY DREAMS

3-inch nub fresh ginger

1 tablespoon honey

1 cup water

Try it this way

Milky: Substitute 1 cup of coconut water for the water.

Green: Add a 2-cup mix of spinach, kale and Romaine lettuce.

Fruity: Add 1 cup of cherries.

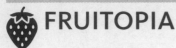 FRUITOPIA

4 sprigs parsley	1 cup strawberries
1 red bell pepper	1 orange
2 tomatoes	½ cup watermelon

Try it this way

Milky: Substitute sprouted grain milk for the watermelon.

Green: Substitute 6 kale leaves, 1 cup of spinach and 1 fennel bulb for the watermelon.

Rooty: Substitute 2 carrots for the watermelon.

LATE-NIGHT REFRESHER

2 fennel bulbs	2 pears
1 apple	½ lemon

Try it this way

Milky: Add ½ cup of brown rice milk.

Green: Add 2 cups of mustard greens.

Rooty: Substitute 1 carrot for the apple.

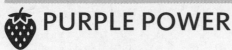 PURPLE POWER

½ head red cabbage

2-inch nub fresh ginger

6 cups Concord grapes

½ cup blackberries

1 Golden Delicious apple

¼ teaspoon ground nutmeg

Try it this way

Milky: Substitute ½ cup of nut milk for half of the grapes.

Green: Substitute 2 cups of Romaine lettuce for half of the red cabbage.

Rooty: Add 2 beets.

WARMING ZEN

½ cucumber

½ cup strawberries

1 tablespoon maple syrup

1 teaspoon ground cinnamon

¼ teaspoon ground nutmeg

1 cup almond milk

Try it this way

Green: Add 5 kale leaves, ¼ wedge of cabbage and ¼ cup of green beans.

Fruity: Add 1 pear and 1 tomato.

Rooty: Add 2 carrots.

WARM MILK

1 tablespoon honey

1 teaspoon ground turmeric

1 cup sprouted grain milk

Try it this way

Green: Add 2 cups of spinach.

Fruity: Add 1 cup of berries.

Rooty: Add 1 small celeriac root.

HOT COCOA

1 tomato

2 tablespoons cocoa powder

1 cup hemp seed milk

Try it this way

Green: Add 1 cabbage head and 5 kale leaves.

Fruity: Add 1 cup of blueberries.

Rooty: Add 2 carrots.

VANILLA CHAI

1-inch nub fresh ginger

¼ teaspoon ground cardamom

1 teaspoon vanilla extract

¼ teaspoon ground cloves

½ teaspoon ground cinnamon

1 cup almond milk

¼ teaspoon ground nutmeg

Try it this way

Green: Add 1 cup of spinach and 1 cup of escarole.

Fruity: Add 1 apple and 1 orange.

Rooty: Add 1 beet and 1 carrot.

THE FINAL SQUEEZE

Here are the answers to seven last questions you probably didn't know you wanted to ask but really, really need to know to get 100 percent juiced.

Q: How do you remove a juice stain from a carpet/shirt/car upholstery?

A: ASAP. Flush the stain with cool water. Sponge (or soak) the stain, using 1 tablespoon of white vinegar mixed with ⅔ cup of rubbing alcohol. Blot until the liquid is absorbed. Leave 15 minutes. Repeat until the stain disappears. Sponge/rinse with water and blot/hang dry.

Q: What's the best thing to do with leftover pulp?

A: Substitute ½ cup of pulp for ¼ cup of flour in any baking recipe or for breadcrumbs in any meatballs/meatloaf/hamburger recipe. Another option is to toss it in soups, stews, oatmeal, smoothies, pancakes, yogurt, sauces, dips or a rice/pasta dish. If you can't use it right away, store it in a baggy and freeze it until ready to use.

Q: I made a fresh quart of juice, then the dog ran out the front door, where my car was getting ticketed. Back inside, the kids were fighting, then I was called to serve the President. Can I really not store my juice?

A: Yes, you should drink your juice ASAP because it's not pasteurized. But life intervenes, so if necessary, store in the back (or coldest) part of the fridge in a glass or stainless steel container filled to the brim (to minimize oxidation) and a splash of lemon juice to help with preservation, and drink within 24 hours (if it tastes strange or the color changes, pour it down the drain). If you must, freeze it in ice cube trays for longer storage but know that this will set back your standing as a Hardcore Juicer by several years.

Q: My juicer broke and I need to juice. Help!

A: Chill, little grasshopper. For the short-term, you can juice using a blender and nut milk bag or some sheets of cheese cloth. Blend the ingredients and pour into the bag, squeezing the pulp to strain the juice into a pitcher. You'll probably need some extra liquid to thin things out.

Q: My juicer keeps jamming.

A: Cut your ingredients smaller. Alternate hard fruits with soft fruits, or fibrous vegetables with non-fibrous vegetables. Set a slow and steady pace when feeding. If it still clogs, try hitting the reverse button for two to three seconds to unblock it, and then continue juicing by switching it to forward again.

Q: What do I do if the juice doesn't press enough liquid?

A: It happens. Add water or one of the liquids from "Get Hydrated" (page 60).
You may have used "dry" ingredients with a low-water content (carrots, peas, broccoli, beets, cabbage, cauliflower, peppers, spinach, raspberries, pineapple, plums, peaches, orange, cranberries, apricots, blueberries, apples, cherries, grapes and pears are all in the lower water range while cucumbers, lettuce, celery, tomatoes, zucchini, watermelons, cantaloupe and grapefruit are high in water).

Q: How can I become a Hardcore Juicer?

A: Juice until at least half of the following apply. You:

○ Worship Dr. Norman Walker, inventor of the first juicer, aka the Norwalk.

○ Have cleansed for three days on just green juices, taken a day off and then rinsed and repeated.

○ Never think it's too early or late to down a juice or make a juice.

○ Crave juice all the time. Seriously. All. The. Time.

○ Lose it if someone accidentally drinks your juice. Big time.

○ Think a kale/cabbage/parsley juice is more refreshing than water.

○ Have permanent green marks on your car seat from traffic spills.

○ Know the best place to buy produce in bulk.

○ Get more excited about kale on sale for 52 cents a pound than you do over winning the lotto.

○ Think fruit in green juice is for wimps.

○ View the beetroot stains on your kitchen counter as badges of cleansing honor.

○ Know exactly which fruit needs peeling without using a cheat sheet.

○ Rarely use a recipe.

○ Own more than one juicer.

○ Know the specs of the few juicers you don't own.

○ Call buying fresh-pressed juice instead of making your own "slumming it."

○ Have an opinion about wheatgrass.

○ Never think steroids when someone says an athlete juices.

○ Would rather gossip about juice entrepreneurs than reality show stars.

○ Can estimate the water content of a cucumber just by hefting it.

INDEX

Afternoon Treat, 147

Alcohol, and cleanse, 79

"All-natural" labeling, 23

All-Purpose Master Green Juice, 127

Aloe vera juice, 60–61

Aloha, 134

Arteries, and cleanse, 92

Arugula, 50

Asparagus, 50, 55

Beach Bum, 161

Beans, 55

Beat It, 133

Beets, 50

Belly Buster, 144

Berries. *See specific berries*

Big Gulp, 170

Big Three, 151

Bitter taste, 46

Blackberries, 56

Bloody Mary, 163

Blue Blood, 162

Blue Moon, 159

Blue/purple-colored produce, 58

Blueberries, 55

Bok choy, 50

Bones, and cleanse, 92–93

Bottles, insulated, 41

Brain, and cleanse, 93

Breakfasts: and cleanse, 100; recipes, 130–36

Brix level, in juice concentrate, 21

Broccoli, 50, 55

Brussels sprouts, 55

Brushes, vegetable, 41

Cabbage, 50

Calories, 82

Candy Apple, 177

Carrot Cake, 172

Carrots, 50

Cauliflower, 50

Centrifugal juicers vs. cold press juicers, 32–34

Chef Salad, 151

Cherry Pie, 177

Cherry Pop, 134

Chocolate Silk, 143

Citric acid, 25

Citrus peelers, 41

Citrus presses, 34

Citrus Squeeze, 157

Cleanses. *See* Juice cleanses

Coco-Nutty, 149

Coconut "Milk" Water, 64

Coconut water, 60

Coffee, and cleanse, 79

Cold press juicers: accessories, 40–42; alternatives, 34–36; benefits, 32–33; shopping tips, 36–40; troubleshooting, 72–75, 187; versatility, 33–34; vs. centrifugal juicers, 32–34

Cold press juicing: basics, 12–29; cleanses, 76–120; defined, 15; equipment, 30–42; FAQs, 186–88; ingredients, 43–75; recipes, 122–85

Colon, and cleanse, 79

Coloring, in bottled juice, 24

Colors, of produce, 58–59

Combinations of produce, 57. *See also* 4:1 ratio

Community Supported Agriculture (CSA), 42

Complex sugars, 20

Compost containers, 42

Concentrate, juice, 21

"Contains real fruit juice" labeling, 22

Cooked vs. raw produce, 49–51

Cookies and Cream, 149

Cooler bags, 42

Corers, 41

Corn sugar, 26

Creamsicle, 145

Cruciferous vegetables, 50. *See also specific vegetables*

Cucumber Spa, 181

Curry Chai, 155

Cutie Pie, 171

Cutting boards, 40

Daily Beast, 168

Date syrup, 61

Day Breaker, 132

Desserts: and cleanse, 102–103; recipes, 174–78

Dinners: and cleanse, 101–102; recipes, 166–73

Dirty Martini, 163

Disaccharides, 20

Drink Your Oats, 136

Dyes, in bottled juice, 24

Energy Boost, 146

Equipment, kitchen, 30–42. *See also* Cold press juicers

Excuses, during cleanse, 88–91

FAQs, 186–88

Fat, healthy, 60

"Fat-free" labeling, 26

Fiber, 16, 59; and cleanse, 83

5x5, 154

Flavonoids, 21

Flavors, of greens, 46

Flour, and cleanse, 79

Fluid intake, 81

Food co-ops, 42
40 Winks, 180
4:1 ratio (fruit to vegetable), 16–18, 57, 74
Fresh vs. frozen produce, 47–48
Fried foods, and cleanse, 79
Frozen vs. fresh produce, 47–48
Fructose, 17, 20
Fruit and vegetable wash, 42
Fruit-flavored drinks, 22
Fruit to vegetable ratio, 16, 18, 74
Fruitier-Tutti, 144
Fruitopia, 182
Fruits: benefits, 12–13. *See also specific fruits*

Galactose, 20
Gardens, 42, 52–56
Garlic, 50
Gastrointestinal tract, and cleanse, 93
Genetically Modified Organisms (GMOs), 25
Gingerbread, 140
Glass straws, 42
Glucose, 20
Glycemic index (GI), 56
Goin' Nutz, 148
The Grass Is Greener, 153
Green Acres, 129
Green Chartreuse, 161
Green-Eyed Monster, 129
Green Goddess, 128
The Green Hulk, 139
Green labels, 25
Green leaf lettuce, 50
Green Meanies, 139
Green-colored produce, 58
"Green Tea," 131
Greens, and flavors, 46
Gut, and cleanse, 93
"Gut scrubbers," 59
"Gut soothers," 60

Happy Dreams, 181
Happy Healthy Herby, 170
Happy hour recipes, 160–65
Hardcore Juicers (HJs), FAQs, 187–88
Hawaiian Punch, 158
Herbs, 54, 60
High starch fruits, 57
Hippy-Dippy Lunch, 156
Home juice bars, 30–42
Hot Cocoa, 184
Hydration, 81
Hydraulic press juicers, 35

In the Green, 128
Ingredients, for cold press juicing, 43–75. *See also* Produce; *see also specific ingredients*
Insulated bottles, 41
Insulin, 20–21
Irradiated foods, 25

Jars, 41
Juice bars, home, 30–42
Juice bars, public, costs, 14
Juice cleanses, 76–120; "cheating," 84–85; contraindications, 87; defined, 76; excuses, 88–91; and health, 91–95; meal plans, 99–103; stages, 96–98; timing, 76–95; types, 103–20
Juice cocktails, 22
Juice drinks, 22
Juicers. *See* Cold press juicers
Juices, bottled, 7, 14–15; labeling, 21–26
Juicing: basics, 43–75; benefits, 7–10, 14–15, 27–29; and cleanse, 76–120; choosing recipes, 43–46; defined, 14; FAQs, 186–88; ingredients, 43–75; moderation, 16–18;

picking produce, 51–65; prepping produce, 66–71; recipes, 122–85; storage, 72, 186–87

"Key" Lime Pie, 178
Kick-Ass Lemonade, 158
Kick in the (Gr)ass, 152
Kick Start, 131
Kidneys, and cleanse, 93
Kissing a Cow, 167
Kitchen Sink, 169
Knives, 40; skills, 68–69
Kombucha tea, 61; recipe, 64–65

Labeling, on bottled juice, 21–26
Lactose, 20
Late-night munchies. *See* Snacks
Late-Night Refresher, 182
Leafy greens, 52
Lemonade, 155
Lettuce keepers, 41
Lettuces, 50, 55
"Lightly sweetened" labeling, 26
Liquid Viagra, 165
Liquids, for juicing, 60–65
Liver, and cleanse, 92
Lunch Combo, 154
Lunches: and cleanse, 101; recipes, 150–59
Lungs, and cleanse, 93–94

"Made with real fruit" labeling, 22
Maltose, 20
Manna, 157
Manual leverage pressers, 34
Mapleberry, 145
Mason jars, 41
Masticating juicers. *See* Cold press juicers
Meal plans, and cleanse, 99–103

Measuring cups, 41
Medical clearance, 10
Medjool Date Syrup, 61
Mega blenders, 34
Menus, sample, 105–106, 110–11, 116–18
Microgreens, 53
Minerals, 24, 59
Mock mochas, 98–99
Mojito, 162
Mold, in bottled juices, 24
Mono juices: menu, 106; recipes, 126–29
Monosaccharides, 20
Mood Indigo, 172
Morning Bracer, 132
Mudslide, 164

"Natural flavors" labeling, 23–24
"Natural" labeling, 23
Neapolitan, 173
"No preservatives" labeling, 24
"No sugar added" labeling, 26
"Not from concentrate" labeling, 22–23
Nut milk bags, 42
Nut/seed milks, 60; recipe, 62

One-Day Quickie Cleansing Plan, 103–108
"100% juice" labeling, 21–22
Onions, 55
Open Sesame, 141
Orange/yellow-colored produce, 58
Organic labeling, 23
Organic vs. conventional produce, 48–49

Pancreas, 20
Paring knives, 40
Pasteurization, of bottled juices, 24–25

Peanut Butter Cup, 138
Peas, 55
Peelers: citrus, 41; vegetable, 40–41
Peppermint Tea, 180
Peppers, 50, 54
Pesticide load, 48–49
Piña Uncolada, 164
Pineapple corers, 41
Pink Drink, 159
PM Pick-Me-Up, 142
Portion sizes, 70–71
Potluck, 169
Pre-cleanse, 116
Presses, citrus, 34
Primary tastes, 45–46
Processed foods, and cleanse, 79
Produce: colors, 58–59; gardening, 52–56; guidelines, 51; picking, 51–65; portion sizes, 70–71; preparation, 66–71; storage, 66–67
Produce bags, reusable, 41
Produce-saver discs, 41
Product labeling, on bottled juice, 21–26
Protein, 59; and cleanse, 85–86
Pulp, 72, 186
Purple/blue-colored produce, 58
Purple Cow, 146
Purple Power, 183

Rainbow juice sample menu, 105
Raspberries, 56
Raw vs. cooked produce, 49–51
Recipes, 122–85; breakfast, 130–36; dessert, 174–78; dinner, 166–73; guidelines, 122–25; happy hour, 160–65; juice types, 124–25; lunch, 150–59; mono

juices, 126–29; snacks, 137–49, 179–85
Red produce, 59
Rice milk, 61; recipe, 63
Rise and Shine, 135
Root vegetables, 53

Salad Bar, 168
Salty taste, 45
Savory taste, 46
Seed/nut milks, 60; recipe, 62
Serving size, of bottled juices, 25
Seven-Day Cleanse That Won't Leave You Starving, 113–20; sample menu, 116–18
Simple sugars, 20
Single-gear juicers. See Cold press juicers
Slap Chops, 42
Slip-ups, while juicing, 74–75
Smurf Juice, 176
Snack Attack, 147
Snacks: and cleanse, 102–103; recipes, 137–49, 179–85
Snickerdoodle, 178
Sodas, sugar content, 17
Solids, and cleanse, 86
Sour taste, 45–46
Sourhead, 175
Soy milk, 61; recipe, 63
Spices, 60
Spicy Mexican Green, 152
Sprouted grain milks, 60; recipe, 62
Sprouters, 42
Sprouts, 53–54
Stages, of cleanse, 96–98
Stains, on cloth, 186
Storage: of juice, 72, 186–87; of produce, 66–67
Strawberries, 55
Strawberry Milkshake, 136
Straws, glass, 42

Strong taste, 46
Sucrose, 20
"Sugar-free" labeling, 26
Sugars, 16–17, 18–21, 26–27; chart, 19; and cleanse, 79; pseudonyms, 27
Sunrise Surprise, 133
Superfoodie, 153
Sweet and Sour, 167
Sweet Greens, 138
Sweet Potato Pie, 143
Sweet Sampler, 142
Sweet taste, 45
Sweeteners, 60. *See also* Sugar
Sweeter than Candy, 148

Tan/white-colored produce, 59
Tastes (sweet, etc.), 45–46

Thermoses, 41
Three-day cleanse sample menu, 110–11
Three-Day Kick-Butt, Belly-Busting, Eat-Less-Crap Cleanse, 108–13
Timetables, for cleanse, 107, 112, 120
Tomatoes, 50–51, 54
Trail Mix, 141
Triturating juicers, 35–36
Tropical Delight, 176
Twilight, 156
Twin-gear juicers, 35–36

Umami, 46
Un-Coffee Frappe, 135

Vanilla Chai, 185
Vegetable brushes, 40
Vegetable peelers, 40–41

Vegetables: benefits, 12–13. *See also specific vegetables*
Veggie Delight, 171
Vitamins, 24, 59

Warm Milk, 184
Warming Zen, 183
Watercress, 50
What's Up Doc?, 140
Wheatgrass, 54
Wheatgrass juicers, 35
White/tan-colored produce, 59

Yellow/orange-colored produce, 58
Yield, 57

Zucchini, 51, 55
Zucchini Cake, 175

ACKNOWLEDGMENTS

Thanks go to Keith Riegert, without whom this book would not have been written, and Alice Riegert, without whom this book would not have been readable!

ABOUT THE AUTHOR

Lisa Sussman has been writing on relationships, health, and careers for over fifteen years. Her book credits include *Green Smoothie Cleanse* (Ulysses Press, 2014), *Am I Weird or Is This Normal?* (Simon and Schuster, 2001), *350 Best Sex Tips Ever* (Carlton, 2002), Sex in the City (Carlton, 2003), *Brazilian Waxes, Lazy Ovaries and Outrageous Orgasms* (Amorata Press, 2005) and *500 Great Dates* (Hearst, 2007). She currently resides in Rhode Island.